*Bite It &*
*Write It !*

## THIS BOOK BELONGS TO

_____

_____

Date journal started on


## NUTRITIONIST'S
## CONTACT INFORMATION

_____

Nutritionist's Name

_____

E-mail

_____

Phone

# Bite It & Write It !

## A GUIDE TO KEEPING TRACK OF WHAT YOU EAT & DRINK

Stacie Castle, RD    Robyn Cotler, RD

Marni Schefter, RD    Shana Shapiro, RD

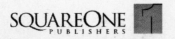

SQUAREONE
PUBLISHERS

COVER DESIGNER: Jeannie Tudor
EDITOR: Colleen Day
TYPESETTER: Terry Wiscovitch
AUTHOR PHOTOS: Jaclyn Fidler
www.jaclynfidlerphotography.com

**Square One Publishers, Inc.**
115 Herricks Road
Garden City Park, New York 11040
(516) 535-2010
(877) 900-BOOK
www.squareonepublishers.com

To learn more about the authors and their work in nutrition:

**Website:** www.biteitandwriteit.com
**Twitter:** @biteitnwriteit
**Facebook:** biteitandwriteit
**Email:** biteitandwriteit@gmail.com

ISBN-13: 978-0-7570-0343-1

Copyright © 2011 by Square One Publishers, Inc.

Printed in the United States of America

10   9   8   7   6   5   4   3   2

# Contents

# Preface

As nutritionists, our job is to help people achieve their dietary goals. Throughout our years of counseling, there is one technique that has consistently resulted in success for our clients: Writing it down. Whether seeking weight loss, disease management, or general wellness, our clients meet their goals more quickly and easily when they keep daily journals of their food consumption and physical activity. The act of writing down meals, snacks, and exercise allows clients to see, and therefore become more aware of, their eating and fitness habits. We, the nutritionists, also benefit from our clients' journals, as they provide us with the details necessary to offer them better care and advice. It is a win-win situation.

Food journals are useful not only for keeping track of *what* you eat, but also for showing *how* you eat. Examining eating behaviors in "black and white" allows more thorough assessments of clients and assists us in setting realistic goals for them. Food journals give us clearer and more holistic pictures of those we counsel, and this in turn allows us to determine which of their eating habits pose the greatest obstacles to their nutritional well-being. Once these behaviors are identified, a personalized plan can be developed to better assist clients in meeting their health goals.

*Bite It and Write It*, which is both a guide and a food journal, is intended to be a tool for clients and practitioners to promote significant dietary and behavioral changes. A collaborative effort of four registered dietitians, this journal's development was made easier by the fact that our clients share many of the same goals. The ten goals presented in this book are the smaller weekly objectives that we have agreed must be met in order to achieve long-term success. We also have a common philosophy when it comes to nutritional practice and counseling: Major behavioral change is achieved when smaller changes are implemented gradually. By focusing on one objective at a time, clients are less overwhelmed and, therefore, more likely to be successful. This is the basic philosophy of *Bite It and Write It*.

Although most of our clients have common *general* goals, we understand that each is also an individual with a unique set of needs. Whether due to diabetes, hypertension, or celiac disease, factors that may need to be monitored greatly vary from client to client. The daily food logs contained in *Bite It and Write It*, although meant for everyone, have also been tailored to meet any specific need a person may have. The logs contain blank columns that can be used for recording sodium intake, carbohydrate counts, or blood glucose values, among other nutritional details.

As nutrition counselors, we also recognize the impact that emotions and other health conditions can have on your weight loss success and overall health. For this reason, the daily food journals in *Bite It and Write It* have a "Notes" section in which feelings or symptoms can be recorded. For instance, if you have irritable bowel syndrome, this space may be useful for writing down any physical symptoms that occur after eating. Frequent binge eaters may want to use this section to write down their emotions prior to or after overeating. All of this information is necessary in order for the client and/or counselor to develop a plan of action.

With *Bite It and Write It*, we have created a journal that puts forth an effective plan for achieving a healthy lifestyle. It is the result of decades of observing firsthand what works for the majority of clients, and each tutorial contains helpful suggestions and "tricks of the trade" to assist you in meeting the weekly goals. In addition, we have included reference tables for calorie counts of some of the most commonly consumed foods, popular restaurant dishes, and concession stand snacks. We hope our effort to provide nutritional guidance in this book is easy-to-follow, beneficial, and a valuable personal and professional tool.

# Introduction

It is as simple as this: Writing down what you eat is the first step towards a healthier lifestyle. People who keep track of their eating and exercise habits lose more weight and keep it off. This is why your food journal is the key to reaching your nutritional and weight loss goals.

Why is a food journal the secret to your success?

• **It makes you accountable.** Being accountable for everything that goes in your mouth makes you more mindful and forces you to think twice before eating.

• **It helps you plan.** Planning meals, snacks, and exercise is essential for maintaining a healthy lifestyle. Whether your goal is to lose weight, tone up, or simply eat healthier, being able to see how much or how little you have eaten and exercised will help you to form weekly goals. You will find that setting smaller goals on a weekly basis achieves lasting results.

• **It pinpoints your problems.** Everyone has personal weaknesses that can stand in the way of weight loss success and optimal health. Keeping a journal will allow you to identify these obstacles more easily and ultimately overcome them.

• **It will keep you motivated.** Writing down your progress and nutritional plan forces you to reflect on your goal, which keeps you focused and determined.

• It assists you in setting realistic goals for yourself. This food journal sets up a ten-week plan that aims at long-term success. Smaller goals will help you focus week to week on what you need to do. Each week, you can reflect on your progress, feel good about your accomplishments, learn from your mistakes, and move forward towards a successful and healthier future.

Although the meaning of "success" varies from one individual to another, there are certain basic rules of nutrition that are necessary for weight loss, disease management, and healthy living in general. This food journal identifies ten goals that, when met, have long-lasting health benefits. In each week of the journal, you will learn how to fulfill a new goal and incorporate it into your daily life. We have included useful tips, information, and charts to aid you in your ten-week journey. At the end of these ten weeks, you will look in the mirror and see a new you.

The journey outlined in *Bite It and Write It* can be fun and exciting, and, at times, frustrating and intimidating. This guide was written to optimize the positive aspects of the journey and alleviate the more difficult ones; it also serves as a way of maintaining a strong commitment to your weight loss and nutrition goals. Use this journal, either independently or with a nutritionist, to track your progress, remain excited and motivated, and ultimately, arrive at your goal.

# How to Use This Book

Few of us really keep track of what we eat. *Bite It and Write It* allows you to record what you eat and drink on a daily basis so that you can better control your diet and reach your personal goals. Think of it as a weekly diary. For ten weeks, we provide a goal for you to focus on for the week, and you in turn will record your progress in attaining that goal. Along the way, we offer vital information, useful tips, and words of inspiration.

## BASIC STEPS TO SUCCESS

Each week of the journal begins with a description of your objective for the next seven days. We believe in taking weight loss one step at a time by setting realistic goals. Setting smaller, realistic goals will make the primary goal—a healthy lifestyle—seem less daunting and unattainable. As you begin this process, keep these four basic steps to success in mind:

**1. Follow our weekly guidelines and goals.** The goals in this journal follow a logical progression, the first few laying the groundwork for the ones that follow. They all lead up to the final goal, which is exercise—an important component in any weight loss plan. If you already exercise, we encourage you to continue throughout the ten weeks; however, if exercise is new to you, we feel that it is best to first master your new eating behaviors before introducing a workout regimen. Of course, some goals will be easier for you to accomplish than others. During the more difficult weeks, try to pinpoint the issues that are standing in the way of your success and then work out a solution. Use the easier weeks to reinforce what you have already achieved, remain determined, and stay on target.

**2. Set your personal goals.** At the end of the weekly goal description, you will find a box in which you will write your own personal goal(s) for that week. Your personal goal should focus on a specific behavior that you will work on changing during the week, which can be decided upon independently or with the assistance of your nutritionist. For example, a weekly goal might be increasing your intake of fruits and vegetables, focusing on portion sizes, or making healthy choices when eating out at a restaurant. After you complete the first week, you will also be able to fill in the section labeled "Weekly Conclusion," which appears directly beneath the "Weekly Personal Goal" section. In the "Weekly Conclusion" space, reflect on the progress made the previous week—your successes, difficulties, and any issues you may still have. Writing down these details allows next week's goals to be shaped and realized.

**3. Track your weight.** On page 16, you will find a chart for recording your weight, which can be a useful quantitative measure of your success. Most people like to track their weight as part of their nutrition regimens, but the frequency varies according to individual needs and preferences. Some check the scale daily; others, weekly; and still others, only with their practitioner. For many people, however, the scale becomes a source of negativity because they begin to obsess over a number rather than focus on health and fitness goals.

It is up to you (and your nutritionist) to decide whether weighing yourself will help or hinder you, and how often it should be done. If you do choose to weigh yourself, write it down in the space provided on the chart each week.

**4. Write in your daily food log.** After each weekly goal, you will find seven daily food logs. This is where you will write it all—the good, the bad, and the ugly. Writing down *everything* will maximize the benefits of this journal.

---

# Ten Ways to Succeed in Healthy Eating

1. Stay positive. Always focus on what you can or *did* do towards achieving your goal, rather than what you didn't do.

2. Stay ahead of the game. Plan and, when possible, prepare snacks and meals ahead of time.

3. Aim for moderation and avoid self-deprivation.

4. Take the time to sit and *enjoy* your food.

5. Eat more often. Eat smaller, appropriately portioned meals and snacks throughout the day—don't save all your calories for one large meal.

6. Learn what your emotional triggers are and how to cope with them without relying on food.

7. Be attuned to your levels of hunger and fullness, and listen to them!

8. Set realistic goals, and allow for bumps in the road. This will keep you moving towards success.

9. Embrace success as a *process*. Gradually implement small changes; don't overwhelm yourself with a complete diet overhaul all at once.

10. Write it down. Keep a well-organized journal to properly manage and account for what you eat.

On the next page is a sample food log. Familiarize yourself with this log so that you understand how to use it properly. Here is a breakdown of each section you will need to fill out:

- **Meals and Snacks.** Fill in each meal and snack in their respective labeled areas. Try to estimate portion size to the best of your ability. To the right of the spaces provided for recording meals, snacks, and their calorie amounts are blank columns that can be used in whatever way best fits your individual needs. For example, if you are trying to lose weight and count calories, you will write down the number of calories in each food consumed. If you have diabetes and need to count carbs, use these blank columns to record the amount of carbohydrates (in grams) that you have eaten at each meal and snack, as well as blood glucose readings. Do you need to manage your blood pressure? Then use this space for keeping track of your sodium intake.

- **Water.** The last column labeled "$H_2O$" contains several boxes, each of which represents eight ounces of water. Every time you drink eight ounces of water, check a box.

- **Exercise.** At the bottom of the log, there is a space in which you can fill in any kind of exercise you did that day and how long you worked out for. Refer to our exercise chart on pages 163 to 164 to calculate how many calories you burn doing various physical activities.

- **Notes.** The area below each meal and snack labeled "Notes" can be used either by you or your nutritionist. Here, write about your hunger and fullness, any physical symptoms you are experiencing, or your emotions. You can also use the space to keep track of when you eat or jot down questions to ask your nutritionist during your next session. This section is intended as a space for you to document and reflect upon your feelings and needs.

## Sample Daily Log

### MONDAY

| | FOOD | CAL. | Carbs | Sodium | | H₂O |
|---|---|---|---|---|---|---|
| **BREAKFAST** | Whole wheat English muffin | 130 | | | | ☑ |
| | 1 egg | 70 | | | | ☑ |
| | 2 egg whites | 40 | | | | |
| | Coffee w/ skim milk | 20 | | | | ☐ |

NOTES: Ask nutritionist about healthy breakfast spreads at next session.

| | | CAL. | | | | |
|---|---|---|---|---|---|---|
| **SNACK** | 1 small apple | 60 | | | | ☑ |
| | 1 tbsp. peanut butter | 95 | | | | ☐ |

NOTES: Hunger rating a 2 before lunch.

| | | CAL. | | | | |
|---|---|---|---|---|---|---|
| **LUNCH** | Chopped salad with 2 oz grilled chicken | 250 | | | | ☑ |
| | 1 tbsp. of balsamic vinegar dressing | 10 | | | | ☑ |
| | 1 small whole grain roll | 110 | | | | ☐ |

NOTES:

| | | CAL. | | | | |
|---|---|---|---|---|---|---|
| **SNACK** | 6 oz yogurt | 90 | | | | ☑ |
| | ½ banana | 50 | | | | ☐ |

NOTES: So hungry for my snack; hunger rating is a 1-2.

| | | CAL. | | | | |
|---|---|---|---|---|---|---|
| **DINNER** | Raw veggies w/ 1 tbsp. hummus | 60 | | | | ☑ |
| | 6 oz grilled salmon | 270 | | | | ☑ |
| | 1 dry baked potato | 145 | | | | |
| | ½ cup of sautéed spinach | 70 | | | | ☐ |

NOTES: Ate dinner around 7, so only hungry for a small snack.

| | | CAL. | | | | |
|---|---|---|---|---|---|---|
| **SNACK** | 1 cup of grapes | 60 | | | | ☐ |

NOTES:

| EXERCISE TYPE | 15 MIN. | 30 MIN. | 45 MIN. | 60 MIN. |
|---|---|---|---|---|
| Running (10 minute mile) | | | ✓ | |

# Hunger/Fullness Awareness Scale

The ultimate purpose of keeping a daily food journal is to become a more mindful eater. This means you should strive to always be aware of how hungry or full you are, and then eat accordingly. Use this scale to rate your levels of hunger and fullness, and record the number in the Notes section of your journal.

**1**

**1. VERY HUNGRY:** This is the most dangerous level to be in, as you probably feel like eating everything in sight. You definitely should have eaten by now in order to stabilize your blood sugar and avoid irritability, anxiety, and lightheadedness.

**2**

**2. READY TO EAT:** Your stomach is growling, and you begin to feel hunger pangs. If you're in this level, you should find something to eat.

**3**

**3. NEUTRAL:** You are neither hungry nor full. Appetite-wise, you feel just right. This is the level of comfort that you should experience between meals.

**4**

**4. SATISFIED:** Ideally, this is the feeling you should have after finishing a properly portioned meal. Be aware that you may not feel immediately satisfied afterwards, especially if you eat too quickly.

**5**

**5. STUFFED:** Danger Zone. We are all familiar with the feeling of being uncomfortably full after a meal—e.g., Thanksgiving. At this level, you are stuffed to the point of sickness and great discomfort.

- **My Hunger/Fullness Awareness Scale.** On the facing page, you will find the Hunger/Fullness Awareness Scale, which we encourage you to reference when writing in the Notes section of journal. Recording your levels of hunger and fullness increases your awareness of your level of satisfaction after each meal, and you may even discover the reasons why you eat in the first place. Sometimes we eat (or overeat) not out of true physical need, but rather out of boredom, emotional reasons, or because the clock indicates that is time to do so. Once you begin paying closer attention to your levels of hunger and fullness, you may find that you have been out of touch with your body's internal signals or unknowingly ignoring them. Before eating, always ask yourself, "Am I really hungry?" You never want to feel uncomfortably stuffed or overly hungry. The key is to eat slowly, eat mindfully, and stop eating when you are satisfied. This way, you will feel and actually *be* in control, and healthier as a result!

## RULES FOR EFFECTIVE JOURNAL USE

We've tried to make it as easy as possible for you to keep a daily food journal. By following a few simple guidelines, you will ensure that your journal is an effective dietary tool.

- **Always write.** It is important that you fill in your log every day. Don't try to record the entire week at once, because you will never remember everything. Details are an essential part of this process and crucial to your success.

- **Be honest.** As important as it is to boost your confidence by writing down your successes, it is even more important to write about the difficulties you encounter. Seeing the poor food choices you've made written down on paper will prompt you to reflect on why you made those choices and prevent you from repeating your mistakes. On the other hand, writing down and re-reading the smart choices you make will raise your self-confidence and keep you motivated. So whether you're having a good day or a bad day, writing about it is a step in the right direction.

● **Tell it all.** The more you write, the more you know. Write down why you eat, how you eat, and where you eat; write about your emotional and physical feelings; even write about the times you have knowingly made mistakes. All of this information is knowledge, and knowledge is truly the key to success.

# Frequently Asked Questions

As nutritionists, we know that our clients have common concerns that are very important to them. Here are ten of the most common questions we get asked, along with the answers. Once you read and understand the information below, you will be in a better position to make smarter decisions about your food choices.

1. How quickly should I be losing weight?

2. What time should I stop eating for the day, and how can I prevent myself from snacking at night?

3. How often should I eat?

4. How can I snack without overeating?

5. Do I need to worry about food combinations?

6. Can I eat Chinese food and sushi?

7. Can I eat frozen yogurt?

8. Can I drink alcohol?

9. Is there a pill I can take to help me lose weight?

10. Do diet drinks, club soda, coffee, and tea count towards my water intake?

**1. How quickly should I be losing weight?** People always want to lose as much weight as they can right away, but healthy weight loss is only $\frac{1}{2}$ pound to 2 pounds per week on average. We say "on average" because weight loss usually fluctuates—some weeks you may lose slightly more weight, and other weeks you may not lose weight at all. Try not to let your weight loss process become an emotional rollercoaster ride by getting discouraged when the pounds don't melt away as quickly as you would like. Instead, focus on the big picture and track your weight loss over a long period of time. Some people may lose more weight initially due to a decrease in water weight (bloat) and then lose smaller amounts as the weeks go on. Remember, if you lose at a healthy rate, you are more likely to maintain your weight loss than if you follow a "get thin quick" diet plan. This is a marathon, not a sprint.

**2. What time should I stop eating for the day, and how can I prevent myself from snacking at night?** The answer to this question varies depending on which weight loss plan you consult, but the fact of the matter is that eating at night is a behavior usually caused by emotions rather than actual hunger. Emotional eating stems from boredom, loneliness, depression, stress, or even relaxation. It is best to eat a sensible dinner and then have a snack at a reasonable hour. If you are someone who gets home later at night, you should still try to eat a portion-controlled dinner and a small snack, and then call it a night. Either way, if you are eating after eight o'clock in the evening, always ask yourself, "Am I hungry?" If the answer is no, then consider a healthier activity that will get your mind off food, such as reading a book, doing a crossword puzzle, calling a friend, or walking on a treadmill. If all else fails, just sit on your hands and breathe!

**3. How often should I eat?** Obviously, not everyone is the same; some people can go a longer period of time without eating than others. As a general rule, you want to eat within the first few hours after you wake up, and then try to eat a meal every four to six hours, and snacks within two to three hours of a meal. This maximizes your metabolism and keeps your blood sugar level stable.

**4. How can I snack without overeating?** Like meals, snacks should be consumed mindfully. There is a definite difference between "snacking" and a *mindful* snack. A mindful snack is one that is portion-controlled, healthy, and can be enjoyed guilt-free. "Snacking" usually has emotional rather than physical triggers, and often involves poor nutritional choices. To snack appropriately, give yourself ten minutes each day to sit down and enjoy something small and nutritious. If you're always on the go, keep a snack bar, small bag of nuts, or piece of fruit with you. Remember, certain snacks can add up calorically quicker than others. Raw veggies and popcorn are lower in calories than chips and cookies.

**5. Do I need to worry about food combinations?** We do not want your meals to become science experiments, but we *do* recommend that you take the time to plan well-balanced meals and snacks. This means that you should be including vegetables and fruits, a carbohydrate, a source of protein, and a small amount of a desirable fat in your meals (and preferably your snacks as well).

**6. Can I eat Chinese food and sushi?** You can eat anywhere and still eat nutritiously. The key is to make healthy choices when dining out at a restaurant (refer to our guide on pages 134 to 137). Everyone needs to enjoy a meal out on occasion, but be smart about what you order.

When ordering food at a Chinese restaurant, we suggest you to stick to steamed meals with sauces ordered on the side. Sushi can be enjoyed without the high-calorie "extras" like spicy sauces, crunchies, and tempura, and you can request less rice or a cucumber wrap. And remember—portion-control!

**7. Can I eat frozen yogurt?** Yes, but don't be fooled into thinking that it is a "free" food—you can't eat it in limitless quantities. Although frozen yogurt can be lower in calories and fat than ice cream, it is not as healthy or nutritious as regular yogurt, and it should not be eaten as a meal replacement. We recommend that you eat a small portion only for an occasional treat and choose a fruit topping over ones that add extra calories, like candy and nuts. Also, remember to account for toppings when you record your frozen yogurt treat in your journal.

**8. Can I drink alcohol?** Yes, but in moderation. There is room for alcohol in your nutritional plan as long as you account for it. There are some drinks that can be high in calories due to mixers (refer to our calorie count for alcohol on page 167). Beverages such as wine, wine spritzers, light beer, and a combination of alcohol (1 ounce), seltzer, and a splash of juice are about a hundred calories per every four ounces. Be sure to include alcoholic drinks in your daily log, be cautious about drink size, and try to limit the number of drinks you have each day. It is recommended that women limit themselves to one alcoholic drink per day, and men, two drinks per day. Although there is research that points to the health benefits of moderate alcohol consumption, this is not a sufficient reason to begin drinking it if you do not already do so.

**9. Is there a pill I can take to help me lose weight?**
Though there are some supplements (whether prescribed or sold in local pharmacies) that may jumpstart weight loss initially, long-term weight loss and maintenance requires lifestyle change. Nothing is worse than losing weight, receiving positive attention from family and friends, and then gaining it all back—plus more—as soon as you stop dieting. Even well-known food delivery diet programs eventually require you to change (unless you plan on eating that food the rest of your life). People who lose weight through one of these methods usually have a more difficult time adjusting to the necessary lifestyle changes than people who embrace change from the beginning. If there really was a magic pill out there, we would tell you.

**10. Do diet drinks, club soda, coffee, and tea count towards my water intake?** This is not an easy question to answer. While the obvious answer may appear to be yes, many of these beverages contain other ingredients that may not be good for you. Some of these liquids can act as diuretics, which increase the loss of your body's water. In addition, drinks that are artificially sweetened may enhance your cravings for carbohydrates, which, of course, can lead to weight gain. Many beverages also contain unnecessary and questionable ingredients such as salt, food coloring, and preservatives. To achieve lasting weight loss and a nutritious lifestyle, the only truly healthy and thirst-satisfying drink is water. Keep in mind that while there are other acceptable drink choices, these should be consumed in moderation and only if your water intake remains at the recommended amount.

# Weight Tracking Chart

This journal does not require you to keep track of the pounds you lose, but doing so may help you gauge your progress. Below is a chart on which you can record your weight loss as you work towards each of the weekly goals. Seeing a lower number on the scale at the end of Week 10 will surely motivate you to continue a healthy, nutritious lifestyle.

START DATE _____     WEIGHT _____

### END OF WEEK 1

| DATE | WEIGHT |
|------|--------|
|      |        |

### END OF WEEK 2

| DATE | WEIGHT |
|------|--------|
|      |        |

### END OF WEEK 3

| DATE | WEIGHT |
|------|--------|
|      |        |

### END OF WEEK 4

| DATE | WEIGHT |
|------|--------|
|      |        |

### END OF WEEK 5

| DATE | WEIGHT |
|------|--------|
|      |        |

### END OF WEEK 6

| DATE | WEIGHT |
|------|--------|
|      |        |

### END OF WEEK 7

| DATE | WEIGHT |
|------|--------|
|      |        |

### END OF WEEK 8

| DATE | WEIGHT |
|------|--------|
|      |        |

### END OF WEEK 9

| DATE | WEIGHT |
|------|--------|
|      |        |

### END OF WEEK 10

| DATE | WEIGHT |
|------|--------|
|      |        |

# Goal 1

## Be Present

**Y**ou may be apprehensive about starting a new nutritional or weight loss plan, and the first week is usually the most difficult. As we explained in the introduction, keeping a food journal is the most effective way to change your eating habits. Food journals force you to pay attention to what you eat, and they remind you of what you have eaten, whether good or bad. So, your first goal is to get in the habit of putting all of your nutritional choices and eating-related behaviors in writing. This will allow you to become more aware of what, why, and how much you eat on a daily basis. In other words, your goal is to become more mentally present before, during, and after meals. Doing so will be *your* best present. For the next ten weeks, strive to be a mindful eater, and you will begin this week by starting—and continuing—this journal.

## WHAT IS MINDFULNESS?

The definition is simple. Being mindful means being aware and present during every moment of your life, including the moments when you are eating. Most people eat and snack without thinking, which often leads to overeating or consuming unhealthy food. When you are mindful of your eating habits, you really pay attention to what you put in your mouth.

# HOW DO YOU BECOME MINDFUL OF YOUR EATING?

There are five ways to increase your eating awareness:

1. Slow down and take a minute to notice your food.

2. Sit down when you eat, and eat slowly. Take the time to enjoy what you are eating.

3. Sense the food. How do the aroma, appearance, texture, and taste of the food make you feel?

4. Pay attention to the amount of food on your plate. Is it appropriately portioned? Do you really need to finish everything on your plate, or will you enjoy your eating experience just as much if you eat only half of it?

5. Know if you are satisfied. Are you enjoying your food? Are you eating until you are satisfied, full, or stuffed?

Mindful eating is really a matter of paying attention—both to what you are eating and how eating it makes you feel. For example, look at an apple. Generally shiny, red, and round, its appearance is pleasing. Bite the apple. It is crunchy, juicy, sweet, and tasty. Now, enjoy the apple. In all likelihood, you feel satisfied rather than full. This is why apples are perfect snacks between meals: Enjoyable and appropriately sized, an apple is a mindful snack.

Mindless eating, however, occurs when you are *not* paying attention: When you go too long without eating and then binge at your next meal to the point of feeling overly stuffed; when you sit down in front of the television after a long day and finish an entire bag of chips without realizing it; when you reach for the breadbasket at a restaurant until there is nothing left to reach for. This type of eating is the kind that can make you overweight and unhealthy.

Very often, mindless eating is a symptom (and a result) of emotional stress. Emotional eating occurs when the desire for food is either knowingly or unknowingly triggered by feelings such as depression, boredom, loneliness, anxiety, or stress rather than true physical need. A person is an emotional eater when food is their way to ignore, suppress, or alleviate these feelings. Whatever the case may be, emotional eating takes thinking out of the eating equation, and this leads to poor food choices and oversized portions. Since physical hunger and fullness are irrelevant to them, emotional eaters find it difficult to stop eating once they start.

A helpful technique you can use to combat emotional eating is to ask the simple question, "Am I really hungry?" If you are eating to ease your emotions, the answer is clearly no. Then, the next question is, "What *am* I hungry for?" This may be the point when you should question whether there is something missing from your life. Oftentimes, people do not need to fill a void, but rather reprioritize their lives. Adjusting priorities can add balance to your life and relieve stress, which is a common trigger for emotional eating. Stress does not magically disappear, so it must be dealt with in a way that does not lead to mindless eating. Food does not cure feelings!

Again, being aware of what and why you eat will allow you to make smarter choices when it comes to food, and writing it down is the first step towards achieving this awareness. When you write down the foods you eat, you immediately become more conscientious of what, when, and how much you are eating. Moreover, writing about your level of hunger, enjoyment of meals, and emotions that cause you to eat will make you more aware of your true feelings, habits, and triggers. Remember, the goal is not to feel stuffed, but satisfied—in both your appetite and your life.

Use the *Bite It and Write It* journal every day. Be honest and share *everything*. Writing in your journal only a couple days a week and including few details suggests that you are not fully committed to your goal. In order to be truly dedicated, you must be willing to tell all (even your weak moments), to be mindful at all times, and to examine the reasons behind your less healthy choices. The more time you spend writing in your journal, the better your results will be.

## WEEKLY PERSONAL GOAL

## WEEKLY CONCLUSION

## MONDAY

| | FOOD | CAL. | | | | H₂O |
|---|---|---|---|---|---|---|
| **BREAKFAST** | | | | | | 🥤 |
| | | | | | | 🥤 |
| | | | | | | 🥤 |

NOTES: _____

| | | | | | | H₂O |
|---|---|---|---|---|---|---|
| **SNACK** | | | | | | 🥤 |
| | | | | | | 🥤 |

NOTES: _____

| | | | | | | H₂O |
|---|---|---|---|---|---|---|
| **LUNCH** | | | | | | 🥤 |
| | | | | | | 🥤 |
| | | | | | | 🥤 |

NOTES: _____

| | | | | | | H₂O |
|---|---|---|---|---|---|---|
| **SNACK** | | | | | | 🥤 |
| | | | | | | 🥤 |

NOTES: _____

| | | | | | | H₂O |
|---|---|---|---|---|---|---|
| **DINNER** | | | | | | 🥤 |
| | | | | | | 🥤 |
| | | | | | | 🥤 |

NOTES: _____

| | | | | | | |
|---|---|---|---|---|---|---|
| **SNACK** | | | | | | 🥤 |

NOTES: _____

| EXERCISE TYPE | 15 MIN. | 30 MIN. | 45 MIN. | 60 MIN. |
|---|---|---|---|---|
| | | | | |

# TUESDAY

| | FOOD | CAL. | | | | H₂O |
|---|---|---|---|---|---|---|
| **BREAKFAST** | | | | | | 🥤 |
| | | | | | | 🥤 |
| | | | | | | 🥤 |
| | | | | | | |

NOTES: _____

| | | | | | | H₂O |
|---|---|---|---|---|---|---|
| **SNACK** | | | | | | 🥤 |
| | | | | | | 🥤 |

NOTES: _____

| | | | | | | |
|---|---|---|---|---|---|---|
| **LUNCH** | | | | | | 🥤 |
| | | | | | | 🥤 |
| | | | | | | 🥤 |
| | | | | | | |

NOTES: _____

| | | | | | | |
|---|---|---|---|---|---|---|
| **SNACK** | | | | | | 🥤 |
| | | | | | | 🥤 |

NOTES: _____

| | | | | | | |
|---|---|---|---|---|---|---|
| **DINNER** | | | | | | 🥤 |
| | | | | | | 🥤 |
| | | | | | | 🥤 |
| | | | | | | |

NOTES: _____

| | | | | | | |
|---|---|---|---|---|---|---|
| **SNACK** | | | | | | 🥤 |

NOTES: _____

| EXERCISE TYPE | 15 MIN. | 30 MIN. | 45 MIN. | 60 MIN. |
|---|---|---|---|---|
| | | | | |

## WEDNESDAY

| | FOOD | CAL. | | | | H₂O |
|---|---|---|---|---|---|---|
| **BREAKFAST** | | | | | | 🥤🥤🥤 |

NOTES: _____

| | FOOD | CAL. | | | | H₂O |
|---|---|---|---|---|---|---|
| **SNACK** | | | | | | 🥤🥤 |

NOTES: _____

| | FOOD | CAL. | | | | H₂O |
|---|---|---|---|---|---|---|
| **LUNCH** | | | | | | 🥤🥤🥤 |

NOTES: _____

| | FOOD | CAL. | | | | H₂O |
|---|---|---|---|---|---|---|
| **SNACK** | | | | | | 🥤🥤 |

NOTES: _____

| | FOOD | CAL. | | | | H₂O |
|---|---|---|---|---|---|---|
| **DINNER** | | | | | | 🥤🥤🥤 |

NOTES: _____

| **SNACK** | | | | | | 🥤 |
|---|---|---|---|---|---|---|

NOTES:

| EXERCISE TYPE | 15 MIN. | 30 MIN. | 45 MIN. | 60 MIN. |
|---|---|---|---|---|
| | | | | |

| THURSDAY | FOOD | CAL. | | | | H₂O |
|---|---|---|---|---|---|---|
| **BREAKFAST** | | | | | | 🥤 |
| | | | | | | 🥤 |
| | | | | | | 🥤 |
| | | | | | | |

NOTES: _____

| **SNACK** | | | | | | 🥤 |
|---|---|---|---|---|---|---|
| | | | | | | 🥤 |

NOTES: _____

| **LUNCH** | | | | | | 🥤 |
|---|---|---|---|---|---|---|
| | | | | | | 🥤 |
| | | | | | | 🥤 |
| | | | | | | |

NOTES: _____

| **SNACK** | | | | | | 🥤 |
|---|---|---|---|---|---|---|
| | | | | | | 🥤 |

NOTES: _____

| **DINNER** | | | | | | 🥤 |
|---|---|---|---|---|---|---|
| | | | | | | 🥤 |
| | | | | | | 🥤 |
| | | | | | | |

NOTES: _____

| **SNACK** | | | | | | 🥤 |
|---|---|---|---|---|---|---|

NOTES: _____

| EXERCISE TYPE | 15 MIN. | 30 MIN. | 45 MIN. | 60 MIN. |
|---|---|---|---|---|
| | | | | |

## FRIDAY

| | FOOD | CAL. | | | | H₂O |
|---|---|---|---|---|---|---|
| **BREAKFAST** | | | | | | 🥛 |
| | | | | | | 🥛 |
| | | | | | | 🥛 |
| | | | | | | |

NOTES: _____

| | | | | | | H₂O |
|---|---|---|---|---|---|---|
| **SNACK** | | | | | | 🥛 |
| | | | | | | 🥛 |

NOTES: _____

| | | | | | | |
|---|---|---|---|---|---|---|
| **LUNCH** | | | | | | 🥛 |
| | | | | | | 🥛 |
| | | | | | | 🥛 |
| | | | | | | |

NOTES: _____

| | | | | | | |
|---|---|---|---|---|---|---|
| **SNACK** | | | | | | 🥛 |
| | | | | | | 🥛 |

NOTES: _____

| | | | | | | |
|---|---|---|---|---|---|---|
| **DINNER** | | | | | | 🥛 |
| | | | | | | 🥛 |
| | | | | | | 🥛 |
| | | | | | | |

NOTES: _____

| **SNACK** | | | | | | 🥛 |
|---|---|---|---|---|---|---|

NOTES: _____

| EXERCISE TYPE | 15 MIN. | 30 MIN. | 45 MIN. | 60 MIN. |
|---|---|---|---|---|
| | | | | |

# SATURDAY

| | FOOD | CAL. | | | | H₂O |
|---|---|---|---|---|---|---|
| **BREAKFAST** | | | | | | |

NOTES: _____

| | | | | | | H₂O |
|---|---|---|---|---|---|---|
| **SNACK** | | | | | | |

NOTES: _____

| | | | | | | H₂O |
|---|---|---|---|---|---|---|
| **LUNCH** | | | | | | |

NOTES: _____

| | | | | | | H₂O |
|---|---|---|---|---|---|---|
| **SNACK** | | | | | | |

NOTES: _____

| | | | | | | H₂O |
|---|---|---|---|---|---|---|
| **DINNER** | | | | | | |

NOTES: _____

| **SNACK** | | | | | |
|---|---|---|---|---|---|

NOTES: _____

| EXERCISE TYPE | 15 MIN. | 30 MIN. | 45 MIN. | 60 MIN. |
|---|---|---|---|---|
| | | | | |

## SUNDAY

| | FOOD | CAL. | | | | H₂O |
|---|---|---|---|---|---|---|
| **BREAKFAST** | | | | | | 🍵 🍵 🍵 |

NOTES: _____

| | | | | | | H₂O |
|---|---|---|---|---|---|---|
| **SNACK** | | | | | | 🍵 🍵 |

NOTES: _____

| | | | | | | H₂O |
|---|---|---|---|---|---|---|
| **LUNCH** | | | | | | 🍵 🍵 🍵 |

NOTES: _____

| | | | | | | H₂O |
|---|---|---|---|---|---|---|
| **SNACK** | | | | | | 🍵 🍵 |

NOTES: _____

| | | | | | | H₂O |
|---|---|---|---|---|---|---|
| **DINNER** | | | | | | 🍵 🍵 🍵 |

NOTES: _____

| | | | | | | H₂O |
|---|---|---|---|---|---|---|
| **SNACK** | | | | | | 🍵 |

NOTES: _____

| EXERCISE TYPE | 15 MIN. | 30 MIN. | 45 MIN. | 60 MIN. |
|---|---|---|---|---|
| | | | | |

# "The Cookie Jar": A Non-Food Activity System

Create a cookie jar at home—but without the cookies! Instead, place single pieces of paper inside the jar. On each piece of paper, write down an activity (not related to food) that can serve as a substitute for a treat. The "cookie jar" technique is especially helpful for emotional eaters. Rather than automatically turn to food, you can pick an activity out of the jar. By replacing mindless eating with fun activities, you will not only discover new ways of relaxing, but also come to understand the difference between boredom and hunger.

Below are ten suggestions for rewards that you can place in your "cookie jar." Be sure to customize the activities to make them relaxing and enjoyable.

1. Call a friend.

2. Read a book.

3. Organize a drawer or closet.

4. Shop online or browse websites for interesting articles and healthy recipes.

5. Buy a new outfit (expensive or inexpensive) that you feel great in.

6. Sit outside and enjoy the fresh air.

7. Go to or rent a movie.

8. Take a walk.

9. Read a magazine, whether it's cooking-related, health-oriented, or a tabloid.

10. Light a candle and *breathe*.

The most difficult part about relaxing without food is that it forces you to make time for *you*. Make the time! You deserve to be your own priority.

# Goal 2
## Keep the Heart of Your Home Healthy

**N**ow that you're in the habit of recording and assessing your food choices, you need to begin taking a closer look at why you often do not make the right ones. If you're like most people, one of the problems is your kitchen, and a kitchen makeover—this week's goal—is the solution.

Last week, you learned how to eat mindfully and become more attuned to your level of satisfaction while eating. This week, you will learn how to organize your kitchen in a way that promotes healthy food choices rather than sabotages your weight loss success. It's time to examine the heart of your home and take the steps necessary to make it healthy.

Begin by looking inside your refrigerator. Are the doors and shelves messy? Is the cookie dough on the top shelf for easy access, while the fruits and vegetables are out of sight, stowed away in the bins below? How many soda cans and bottles do you see? After you give it the once-over, begin emptying everything out.

Next, check out your pantry. Is it overflowing with snacks? Is it littered with crumb-filled bags and containers? How many appealing *and* healthy choices does your pantry offer? Probably not enough—so, once again, empty it out.

# IT BEGINS IN YOUR KITCHEN

Follow these ten steps to perfect your kitchen makeover:

**1.** Wipe the refrigerator door and shelves with a mixture of water and white vinegar.

**2.** Organize your food by category. Look at your clean, empty refrigerator and visualize where foods should be placed.

**3.** Display the fruits and vegetables intended for snacking at eye level. They should be on the top shelf so that when you open the door, they are the first thing you see and the easiest to grab. Take them out of the bags, wash them, and put them in bowls, or cut them up to store in plastic containers. Chopped fruit is a quick and easy healthy snack, and the more colorful the fruit assortment is, the more appetizing it will be.

**4.** Clear a space for dairy products. Arrange yogurts, cheeses, and hard-boiled eggs on the same shelf, along with seeds, nuts, and nut butters (nuts go rancid quickly and will last longer in the refrigerator). Milk should be stored on a lower shelf because you will always find it regardless of its location.

**5.** Place high-fiber breads and healthy leftovers next to each other. It is helpful to have appetizing *and* healthy prepared foods readily available so that you won't be tempted to eat less nutritious food out of pure laziness.

**6.** Vegetables being used for cooking can be stored in the drawers as well as foods that must be consumed less frequently and kept out of sight, such as pudding and soda.

**7.** Put all of your sauces, dressings, and condiments in the door shelves. Make sure that they fit within nutritional guidelines and have not expired. It also helps to have a wide and healthy variety.

**8.** Don't forget the freezer: Throw away anything that's been in there too long. Leave frozen vegetables and fruits in the door in plain sight, mark your leftovers, and organize your meats. Keep healthy breads, muffins, and breakfast foods together. Ice cream and treats should be placed in drawers—out of sight, out of mind.

**9.** Your pantry also needs a renovation. Empty and wash down all the shelves before replacing the food. Toss the foods

---

## Keep It Clean!

A clean kitchen is the perfect home for your healthy food, but you must remember to use only safe and sanitary cleaning methods. The safety recommendations of chemicals found in various cleaning products change regularly, and the kitchen is one area where you can't take any chances. Here is the safest, cheapest way that you can wipe down your refrigerator and freezer shelves—D.I.Y. (Do It Yourself)!

**You will need:**

❑ An empty spray bottle
❑ Water
❑ White vinegar

**Preparation:**

Mix ⅔ cups of water with ⅓ cups of white vinegar in your spray bottle. Shake it, and you have made a fabulous, effective, and most importantly, *safe* cleaning solution.

---

*Note:* If you prefer to purchase a cleaner, Seventh Generation and Mrs. Meyer's are both safe and eco-friendly. We also recommend Windex Multi-Surface with vinegar for cleaning glass shelves and stainless steel doors. Wood shelves can be wiped down with a rag soaked in soapy water.

that will sabotage your weight loss success or are simply not healthy choices. Measure appropriately sized portions of whole grain crackers or other acceptable snack foods and store them in small plastic bags or containers. If you find it difficult to limit yourself to ten chips, purchase smaller or single serving bags instead. Again, healthier snacks should be placed at eye level, and treats stored on the top shelf or another place that is not visible.

**10.** If you see it, you eat it. Therefore, only fruit should remain on the counter. Cookies, candy, cake, and pretzels should never be left out—they will only lead to mindless snacking.

## PORTION CONTROL: LESS IS MORE

Now that you have committed yourself to mindful eating by keeping a food journal and revamping your refrigerator, the next step is to pay closer attention to *how much* you are eating. As a society, we have become accustomed to large portions, and most people want to get their "money's worth" when buying food or dining out. You probably expect to be served a large plate filled with food at a restaurant, and you might even complain if a less generous portion is placed in front of you. You look to get more "bang for your buck" when buying bagels at the local shop—each of which is the equivalent of six slices of bread. You might even fall into common fast food chain traps, as many places now offer super-sized specials that entice you to buy more food at a lower price. While these kinds of bargains are indeed giving you your "money's worth," they can also make you overweight.

Society is not responsible for watching your waistline, so it is up to you to know correct portion sizes and eat accordingly. When you are not eating mindfully, you unknowingly consume large quantities of food simply because it is there in front of you, not because you need a large amount to feel satisfied and enjoy your eating experience. Eating mindfully requires you to consider not only what you are consuming, but how much.

Here are some more general rules you should follow when portioning your food:

• **Use a smaller plate.** A smaller plate makes portions appear larger (and therefore, more satisfying), so you will eat less.

• **Never eat out of a bag or container.** Measure properly sized portions of foods that are sold in large containers or bags. You can even store servings of certain foods—nuts, for example—in small plastic bags for a ready-made snack on the go. Check out our Nut Portion Guide on page 129.

• **Bulk your portions with veggies.** Increasing the volume of your recommended portions with vegetables will keep you more satisfied. Adding mixed vegetables to ½ cup of pasta, for instance, can help fill your plate *and* your stomach.

• **Don't be a member of the "Clean Plate Club."** Since portion sizes are usually too large at restaurants, always pay attention to how much food is placed in front of you, and then try to visualize a more appropriate serving. Rather than finish everything on your plate, offer to share your meal or bring some home with you.

• **Read food labels.** The inset on pages 42 to 44 features a sample food label. Notice the specified *serving size*. You should note *how many servings* make up that package before you consume it. Nowadays, many food items are sold in individual servings or smaller packages. If you have a problem limiting yourself when it comes to certain foods, you may benefit from purchasing smaller packages or measuring portions into smaller plastic bags to store in your pantry.

Notice the difference in your eating habits when you begin to consider portion size in a reorganized kitchen that promotes healthy eating. You can maintain your kitchen makeover by cleaning out the refrigerator, pantry, and cabinets each month and replenishing them with healthy food items each week. Congratulate yourself for creating an environment that will enable you to achieve the healthy lifestyle that you want.

## WEEKLY PERSONAL GOAL

_____

_____

_____

_____

_____

_____

## WEEKLY CONCLUSION

_____

_____

_____

_____

_____

_____

## MONDAY

| | FOOD | CAL. | | | | H₂O |
|---|---|---|---|---|---|---|
| **BREAKFAST** | | | | | | 🥤 |
| | | | | | | 🥤 |
| | | | | | | 🥤 |

NOTES: _____

| | FOOD | CAL. | | | | H₂O |
|---|---|---|---|---|---|---|
| **SNACK** | | | | | | 🥤 |
| | | | | | | 🥤 |

NOTES: _____

| | FOOD | CAL. | | | | H₂O |
|---|---|---|---|---|---|---|
| **LUNCH** | | | | | | 🥤 |
| | | | | | | 🥤 |
| | | | | | | 🥤 |

NOTES: _____

| | FOOD | CAL. | | | | H₂O |
|---|---|---|---|---|---|---|
| **SNACK** | | | | | | 🥤 |
| | | | | | | 🥤 |

NOTES: _____

| | FOOD | CAL. | | | | H₂O |
|---|---|---|---|---|---|---|
| **DINNER** | | | | | | 🥤 |
| | | | | | | 🥤 |
| | | | | | | 🥤 |

NOTES: _____

| **SNACK** | | | | | | 🥤 |
|---|---|---|---|---|---|---|

NOTES: _____

| EXERCISE TYPE | | 15 MIN. | 30 MIN. | 45 MIN. | 60 MIN. |
|---|---|---|---|---|---|
| | | | | | |

## TUESDAY

| | FOOD | CAL. | | | | H₂O |
|---|---|---|---|---|---|---|
| **BREAKFAST** | | | | | | 🥤 |
| | | | | | | 🥤 |
| | | | | | | 🥤 |
| | | | | | | |

NOTES: _____

| | FOOD | CAL. | | | | H₂O |
|---|---|---|---|---|---|---|
| **SNACK** | | | | | | 🥤 |
| | | | | | | 🥤 |

NOTES: _____

| | FOOD | CAL. | | | | H₂O |
|---|---|---|---|---|---|---|
| **LUNCH** | | | | | | 🥤 |
| | | | | | | 🥤 |
| | | | | | | 🥤 |
| | | | | | | |

NOTES: _____

| | FOOD | CAL. | | | | H₂O |
|---|---|---|---|---|---|---|
| **SNACK** | | | | | | 🥤 |
| | | | | | | 🥤 |

NOTES: _____

| | FOOD | CAL. | | | | H₂O |
|---|---|---|---|---|---|---|
| **DINNER** | | | | | | 🥤 |
| | | | | | | 🥤 |
| | | | | | | 🥤 |
| | | | | | | |

NOTES: _____

| **SNACK** | | | | | 🥤 |
|---|---|---|---|---|---|

NOTES: _____

| EXERCISE TYPE | 15 MIN. | 30 MIN. | 45 MIN. | 60 MIN. |
|---|---|---|---|---|
| | | | | |

## WEDNESDAY

| | FOOD | CAL. | | | | H₂O |
|---|------|------|---|---|---|-----|
| **BREAKFAST** | | | | | | 🍵 |
| | | | | | | 🍵 |
| | | | | | | 🍵 |
| | | | | | | |

NOTES: _____

| | | CAL. | | | | H₂O |
|---|---|------|---|---|---|-----|
| **SNACK** | | | | | | 🍵 |
| | | | | | | 🍵 |

NOTES: _____

| | | CAL. | | | | H₂O |
|---|---|------|---|---|---|-----|
| **LUNCH** | | | | | | 🍵 |
| | | | | | | 🍵 |
| | | | | | | 🍵 |

NOTES: _____

| | | CAL. | | | | H₂O |
|---|---|------|---|---|---|-----|
| **SNACK** | | | | | | 🍵 |
| | | | | | | 🍵 |

NOTES: _____

| | | CAL. | | | | H₂O |
|---|---|------|---|---|---|-----|
| **DINNER** | | | | | | 🍵 |
| | | | | | | 🍵 |
| | | | | | | 🍵 |

NOTES: _____

| | | CAL. | | | | H₂O |
|---|---|------|---|---|---|-----|
| **SNACK** | | | | | | 🍵 |

NOTES: _____

| EXERCISE TYPE | 15 MIN. | 30 MIN. | 45 MIN. | 60 MIN. |
|---------------|---------|---------|---------|---------|
| | | | | |

## THURSDAY

| | FOOD | CAL. | | | | H₂O |
|---|---|---|---|---|---|---|
| **BREAKFAST** | | | | | | 🥤 |
| | | | | | | 🥤 |
| | | | | | | 🥤 |

NOTES: _____

| | | | | | | H₂O |
|---|---|---|---|---|---|---|
| **SNACK** | | | | | | 🥤 |
| | | | | | | 🥤 |

NOTES: _____

| | | | | | | |
|---|---|---|---|---|---|---|
| **LUNCH** | | | | | | 🥤 |
| | | | | | | 🥤 |
| | | | | | | 🥤 |

NOTES: _____

| | | | | | | |
|---|---|---|---|---|---|---|
| **SNACK** | | | | | | 🥤 |
| | | | | | | 🥤 |

NOTES: _____

| | | | | | | |
|---|---|---|---|---|---|---|
| **DINNER** | | | | | | 🥤 |
| | | | | | | 🥤 |
| | | | | | | 🥤 |

NOTES: _____

| | | | | | | |
|---|---|---|---|---|---|---|
| **SNACK** | | | | | | 🥤 |

NOTES: _____

| EXERCISE TYPE | | 15 MIN. | 30 MIN. | 45 MIN. | 60 MIN. |
|---|---|---|---|---|---|
| | | | | | |

# FRIDAY

| | FOOD | CAL. | | | | H₂O |
|---|---|---|---|---|---|---|
| **BREAKFAST** | | | | | | 🥤 |
| | | | | | | 🥤 |
| | | | | | | 🥤 |
| | | | | | | |

NOTES: _____

| | | | | | | H₂O |
|---|---|---|---|---|---|---|
| **SNACK** | | | | | | 🥤 |
| | | | | | | 🥤 |

NOTES: _____

| | | | | | | H₂O |
|---|---|---|---|---|---|---|
| **LUNCH** | | | | | | 🥤 |
| | | | | | | 🥤 |
| | | | | | | 🥤 |
| | | | | | | |

NOTES: _____

| | | | | | | H₂O |
|---|---|---|---|---|---|---|
| **SNACK** | | | | | | 🥤 |
| | | | | | | 🥤 |

NOTES: _____

| | | | | | | H₂O |
|---|---|---|---|---|---|---|
| **DINNER** | | | | | | 🥤 |
| | | | | | | 🥤 |
| | | | | | | 🥤 |
| | | | | | | |

NOTES: _____

| **SNACK** | | | | | | 🥤 |
|---|---|---|---|---|---|---|

NOTES: _____

| EXERCISE TYPE | | 15 MIN. | 30 MIN. | 45 MIN. | 60 MIN. |
|---|---|---|---|---|---|
| | | | | | |

## SATURDAY

| | FOOD | CAL. | | | | H₂O |
|---|---|---|---|---|---|---|
| **BREAKFAST** | | | | | | |

NOTES: _____

| | | | | | | H₂O |
|---|---|---|---|---|---|---|
| **SNACK** | | | | | | |

NOTES: _____

| | | | | | | H₂O |
|---|---|---|---|---|---|---|
| **LUNCH** | | | | | | |

NOTES: _____

| | | | | | | H₂O |
|---|---|---|---|---|---|---|
| **SNACK** | | | | | | |

NOTES: _____

| | | | | | | H₂O |
|---|---|---|---|---|---|---|
| **DINNER** | | | | | | |

NOTES: _____

| **SNACK** | | | | | | |
|---|---|---|---|---|---|---|

NOTES: _____

| EXERCISE TYPE | 15 MIN. | 30 MIN. | 45 MIN. | 60 MIN. |
|---|---|---|---|---|
| | | | | |

# SUNDAY

| | FOOD | CAL. | | | | H₂O |
|---|---|---|---|---|---|---|
| **BREAKFAST** | | | | | | 🥤 |
| | | | | | | 🥤 |
| | | | | | | 🥤 |
| | | | | | | |

NOTES:

| | | | | | | H₂O |
|---|---|---|---|---|---|---|
| **SNACK** | | | | | | 🥤 |
| | | | | | | 🥤 |

NOTES:

| | | | | | | H₂O |
|---|---|---|---|---|---|---|
| **LUNCH** | | | | | | 🥤 |
| | | | | | | 🥤 |
| | | | | | | 🥤 |
| | | | | | | |

NOTES:

| | | | | | | H₂O |
|---|---|---|---|---|---|---|
| **SNACK** | | | | | | 🥤 |
| | | | | | | 🥤 |

NOTES:

| | | | | | | H₂O |
|---|---|---|---|---|---|---|
| **DINNER** | | | | | | 🥤 |
| | | | | | | 🥤 |
| | | | | | | 🥤 |
| | | | | | | |

NOTES:

| **SNACK** | | | | | | 🥤 |
|---|---|---|---|---|---|---|

NOTES:

| EXERCISE TYPE | 15 MIN. | 30 MIN. | 45 MIN. | 60 MIN. |
|---|---|---|---|---|
| | | | | |

# How to Read a Food Label

Nutrition labels provide the information necessary to make an educated decision about what foods should be in your refrigerator, your pantry, and ultimately, your body. Use the sample below, along with our tips, to help guide you through the process of reading and comprehending a food label. It may seem overwhelming at first, but once you understand the listed information, you'll find food labels a valuable tool both at home and in the supermarket.

**1. Look at the serving size and the number of servings per package.** Ask yourself, "How many servings am I consuming?" The number of servings you eat determines the number of calories and amount of nutrients you consume. In the label above, a single serving of macaroni and cheese is one cup. Since one box of macaroni and cheese contains two servings, you would consume two cups, and twice as many calories and nutrients, if you ate an entire package.

**2. After determining the serving size, look at the calories.** Calories measure how much energy is contained in a single serving of a particular food. Appropriate calorie amounts vary depending on whether a given food is intended as a meal (300 to 600 calories), a side dish (100 to 250 calories), or a snack (100 to 200 calories).

**3. Focus on important nutrients.** Once you know how many calories are in a serving, notice how much fiber, protein, or carbohydrates are in the food depending on what your specific needs are. If the food is a grain (breads, cereals, pasta, and rice), make sure that it contains a sufficient amount of fiber (5 grams or more per

**Sample Nutritional Label
for Macaroni and Cheese**

# Nutrition Facts

**Begin
Here**

Serving Size 1 cup (228g)
Servings Per Container 2

Amount Per Serving

| Calories 250 | Calories from Fat 110 |
|---|---|

% Daily Value*

**Limit
these
Nutrients**

| | |
|---|---|
| Total Fat 12g | 18% |
| Saturated Fat 3g | 15% |
| Trans Fat 1.5g | |
| Cholesterol 30mg | 10% |
| Sodium 470mg | 20% |
| Total Carbohydrate 31g | 10% |
| Dietary Fiber 0g | 0% |
| Sugars 5g | |
| Protein 5g | |

**Quick
Guide
to % DV**

5% or less
is low

20% or more
is high

**Get
Enough
of these
Nutrients**

| | |
|---|---|
| Vitamin A | 4% |
| Vitamin C | 2% |
| Calcium | 20% |
| Iron | 4% |

**Footnote**

*Percent Daily Values are based on a 2,000 calorie diet.
Your Daily Values may be higher or lower depending on
your calorie needs:

| | Calories: | 2,000 | 2,500 |
|---|---|---|---|
| Total Fat | Less than | 65g | 80g |
| Sat Fat | Less than | 20g | 25g |
| Cholesterol | Less than | 300mg | 300mg |
| Sodium | Less than | 2,400mg | 2,400mg |
| Total Carbohydrate | | 300g | 375g |
| Dietary Fiber | | 25g | 30g |

serving is ideal). *Always* choose whole grains over refined grains and flours. Look for bread products with labels that say *whole grain, whole wheat, rye,* and *oatmeal.* You will know if a food is made from refined grains if the label says *cracked wheat, made with whole grain, made with whole wheat, multi-grain,* or *oat bran.*

**4. Know what to avoid.** Limit the amount of saturated fat in your food. Compare different brands of the same product and buy the one that contains the least amount of saturated fat. In addition, the American Heart Association now recommends no more than 1,500 mg of sodium per day instead of 2,000 mg, which is the amount listed on food labels. Control how much sodium you consume on a daily basis and cut out trans fats as much as possible.

**5. Understand Percent Daily Values (%DV).** Daily Value recommendations for key nutrients are based on a 2,000-calorie daily diet. To figure out how nutrient-rich the food is, pay attention to the listed percentages: Anything less than 5 percent is insignificant, and more than 20 percent is plentiful. Keep in mind that if you consume more than 2,000 calories a day, the Percent Daily Values are not applicable.

**6. Note the footnote.** The table directly underneath the %DV recommendations lists the daily minimum and maximum requirements for certain nutrients based on 2,000- and 2,500-calorie diets. These amounts remain the same on every product, which distinguishes the table from Percent Daily Values. Daily requirements for fat, cholesterol, sodium, carbohydrates, and dietary fiber do *not* change.

# Goal 3
## Shop for Food Like a Pro

Last week, you were introduced to nutrition labels and learned how to read and analyze them proficiently. This knowledge is a basic part of "shopping smart," and you will quickly realize its value the next time you are in the supermarket, if you haven't already. Shopping smartly, efficiently, and healthfully is essential if you want a healthy lifestyle, and it is your goal for this week. Knowing how to read a nutrition label once you're in the grocery store is only half the battle; planning and preparing your weekly trip there is just as crucial. Below are some suggestions for making your next supermarket visit productive and nutritious.

• **Before leaving your house, take an inventory of your kitchen.** To ensure that you only buy what you need, thoroughly inspect your pantry and refrigerator first. *Write down* every food that needs to be purchased and restocked.

• **Plan your meals ahead of time.** Buy a week's worth of breakfast ingredients and at least four nights of dinner ingredients each time you go food shopping. Plan out quick and easy lunches to avoid letting purchased food items go to waste.

• **Arm yourself with a list.** Bringing and sticking to your shopping list is another effective way to prevent yourself from buying food impulsively. Refer to the *Bite It and Write It* shopping guide on pages 56 to 60 for a comprehensive list of the kinds of foods you should buy.

- **Never grocery shop while hungry.** Shopping on an empty stomach will only lead to unhealthy snacks and other food items being carelessly tossed in your cart.

- **Shop the perimeter.** Most supermarkets have similar layouts. The produce, dairy, and meat, poultry, and fish sections

## From Hand to Mouth

Determining correct serving sizes can be tricky and confusing, so using your own hand to measure portion sizes is a good rule of thumb (pun intended). The guide below is meant to *give you a hand* in measuring proper portions for various foods.

| PORTION | HAND | EXAMPLES |
| --- | --- | --- |
| 1 teaspoon | Tip of thumb | Oil, butter, sugar, mayonnaise |
| 1 tablespoon | ½ thumb | Honey, ketchup |
| 2 tablespoons | Whole thumb | Salad dressing, nut butter, grated cheese, dried fruit |
| ¼ cup | 1 hand cupped | Beans, hummus, guacamole |
| 4 oz. or ½ cup | Palm of hand or 1 open handful | Fish, turkey, chicken, beef, pork, burgers, pasta, rice, fruit salad, melon, grapes |
| 1 cup | Whole fist | Cereal, medium fruit, berries, vegetables, yogurt, soup, chili, chips |

are set up along the perimeter of the store, while the aisles are typically filled with processed foods. The majority of the foods you buy should come from the periphery. Venture to the middle aisles only for items that you really need.

• **Go heavy on fresh produce.** When you can, purchase pre-cut fruits and vegetables, since you're more likely to eat healthy when not as much effort is required. Alternatively, plan to clean and chop up your produce as soon as you get home (while you're still motivated).

• **Go light on packaged snack foods.** There is very little need for these foods in your diet or your life in general. If you are a parent and feel you need to buy snacks for your kids, purchase ones that are healthy and will not tempt you. It goes without saying that you should limit the amount you buy.

• **Spice it up.** Start getting in the habit of buying herbs and spices to enhance the taste of your meals, as these are healthy, low-calorie alternatives to the oils and dressings that are more commonly used to flavor cuisine. Be adventurous and try to add herbs and spices to everyday recipes: Fresh dill can be added to a garden or chicken salad, curry tastes great on roasted cauliflower, and a sprinkling of cinnamon in your oatmeal or butternut squash really makes a difference. Many herbs and spices also offer numerous health benefits. For example, cinnamon helps to control blood sugar, and turmeric (or curcumin) has anti-tumor properties. If you are unsure of what sp' should be added to different foods, you car ' (preferably without salt), which is a m' herbs and spices. Rubs are sold in mo packages usually tell you which foo used to flavor.

If you use these tips as well as our pre-printed food shopping list, you will be well on your way to becoming an informed, mindful, and nutritious shopper in the supermarket.

## WEEKLY PERSONAL GOAL

## WEEKLY CONCLUSION

## MONDAY

| | FOOD | CAL. | | | | H₂O |
|---|---|---|---|---|---|---|
| **BREAKFAST** | | | | | | 🍵 |
| | | | | | | 🍵 |
| | | | | | | 🍵 |
| | | | | | | |

NOTES: _____

| | | | | | | H₂O |
|---|---|---|---|---|---|---|
| **SNACK** | | | | | | 🍵 |
| | | | | | | 🍵 |

NOTES: _____

| | | | | | | H₂O |
|---|---|---|---|---|---|---|
| **LUNCH** | | | | | | 🍵 |
| | | | | | | 🍵 |
| | | | | | | 🍵 |
| | | | | | | |

NOTES: _____

| | | | | | | H₂O |
|---|---|---|---|---|---|---|
| **SNACK** | | | | | | 🍵 |
| | | | | | | 🍵 |

NOTES: _____

| | | | | | | H₂O |
|---|---|---|---|---|---|---|
| **DINNER** | | | | | | 🍵 |
| | | | | | | 🍵 |
| | | | | | | 🍵 |
| | | | | | | |

NOTES: _____

| | | | | | | |
|---|---|---|---|---|---|---|
| **SNACK** | | | | | | 🍵 |

NOTES: _____

| EXERCISE TYPE | 15 MIN. | 30 MIN. | 45 MIN. | 60 MIN. |
|---|---|---|---|---|
| | | | | |

| TUESDAY | FOOD | CAL. | | | | H₂O |
|---------|------|------|---|---|---|-----|
| **BREAKFAST** | | | | | | 🥛 |
| | | | | | | 🥛 |
| | | | | | | 🥛 |
| | | | | | | |

NOTES:

| **SNACK** | | | | | | 🥛 |
|-----------|---|---|---|---|---|-----|
| | | | | | | 🥛 |

NOTES:

| **LUNCH** | | | | | | 🥛 |
|-----------|---|---|---|---|---|-----|
| | | | | | | 🥛 |
| | | | | | | 🥛 |
| | | | | | | |

NOTES:

| **SNACK** | | | | | | 🥛 |
|-----------|---|---|---|---|---|-----|
| | | | | | | 🥛 |

NOTES:

| **DINNER** | | | | | | 🥛 |
|-----------|---|---|---|---|---|-----|
| | | | | | | 🥛 |
| | | | | | | 🥛 |
| | | | | | | |

NOTES:

| **SNACK** | | | | | 🥛 |
|-----------|---|---|---|---|-----|

NOTES:

| EXERCISE TYPE | 15 MIN. | 30 MIN. | 45 MIN. | 60 MIN. |
|---------------|---------|---------|---------|---------|
| | | | | |

# WEDNESDAY

| | FOOD | CAL. | | | | H₂O |
|---|---|---|---|---|---|---|
| **BREAKFAST** | | | | | | 🥤 |
| | | | | | | 🥤 |
| | | | | | | 🥤 |

NOTES: _____

| | FOOD | CAL. | | | | H₂O |
|---|---|---|---|---|---|---|
| **SNACK** | | | | | | 🥤 |
| | | | | | | 🥤 |

NOTES: _____

| | FOOD | CAL. | | | | H₂O |
|---|---|---|---|---|---|---|
| **LUNCH** | | | | | | 🥤 |
| | | | | | | 🥤 |
| | | | | | | 🥤 |

NOTES: _____

| | FOOD | CAL. | | | | H₂O |
|---|---|---|---|---|---|---|
| **SNACK** | | | | | | 🥤 |
| | | | | | | 🥤 |

NOTES: _____

| | FOOD | CAL. | | | | H₂O |
|---|---|---|---|---|---|---|
| **DINNER** | | | | | | 🥤 |
| | | | | | | 🥤 |
| | | | | | | 🥤 |

NOTES: _____

| | | | | | | |
|---|---|---|---|---|---|---|
| **SNACK** | | | | | | 🥤 |

NOTES: _____

| EXERCISE TYPE | | 15 MIN. | 30 MIN. | 45 MIN. | 60 MIN. |
|---|---|---|---|---|---|
| | | | | | |

| THURSDAY | FOOD | CAL. | | | | H₂O |
|---|---|---|---|---|---|---|
| **BREAKFAST** | | | | | | 🥛 |
| | | | | | | 🥛 |
| | | | | | | 🥛 |
| | | | | | | |

NOTES:

| **SNACK** | | | | | | 🥛 |
|---|---|---|---|---|---|---|
| | | | | | | 🥛 |

NOTES:

| **LUNCH** | | | | | | 🥛 |
|---|---|---|---|---|---|---|
| | | | | | | 🥛 |
| | | | | | | 🥛 |
| | | | | | | |

NOTES:

| **SNACK** | | | | | | 🥛 |
|---|---|---|---|---|---|---|
| | | | | | | 🥛 |

NOTES:

| **DINNER** | | | | | | 🥛 |
|---|---|---|---|---|---|---|
| | | | | | | 🥛 |
| | | | | | | 🥛 |
| | | | | | | |

NOTES:

| **SNACK** | | | | | | 🥛 |
|---|---|---|---|---|---|---|

NOTES:

| EXERCISE TYPE | 15 MIN. | 30 MIN. | 45 MIN. | 60 MIN. |
|---|---|---|---|---|
| | | | | |

# FRIDAY

| | FOOD | CAL. | | | | H₂O |
|---|---|---|---|---|---|---|
| **BREAKFAST** | | | | | | 🥤 |
| | | | | | | 🥤 |
| | | | | | | 🥤 |
| | | | | | | |

NOTES: _____

| | FOOD | CAL. | | | | H₂O |
|---|---|---|---|---|---|---|
| **SNACK** | | | | | | 🥤 |
| | | | | | | 🥤 |

NOTES: _____

| | FOOD | CAL. | | | | H₂O |
|---|---|---|---|---|---|---|
| **LUNCH** | | | | | | 🥤 |
| | | | | | | 🥤 |
| | | | | | | 🥤 |

NOTES: _____

| | FOOD | CAL. | | | | H₂O |
|---|---|---|---|---|---|---|
| **SNACK** | | | | | | 🥤 |
| | | | | | | 🥤 |

NOTES: _____

| | FOOD | CAL. | | | | H₂O |
|---|---|---|---|---|---|---|
| **DINNER** | | | | | | 🥤 |
| | | | | | | 🥤 |
| | | | | | | 🥤 |

NOTES: _____

| | | | | | H₂O |
|---|---|---|---|---|---|
| **SNACK** | | | | | 🥤 |

NOTES: _____

| EXERCISE TYPE | 15 MIN. | 30 MIN. | 45 MIN. | 60 MIN. |
|---|---|---|---|---|
| | | | | |

# SATURDAY

| | FOOD | CAL. | | | | H$_2$O |
|---|---|---|---|---|---|---|
| **BREAKFAST** | | | | | | |
| | | | | | | |
| | | | | | | |
| | | | | | | |

NOTES:

| | FOOD | CAL. | | | | H$_2$O |
|---|---|---|---|---|---|---|
| **SNACK** | | | | | | |
| | | | | | | |

NOTES:

| | FOOD | CAL. | | | | H$_2$O |
|---|---|---|---|---|---|---|
| **LUNCH** | | | | | | |
| | | | | | | |
| | | | | | | |

NOTES:

| | FOOD | CAL. | | | | H$_2$O |
|---|---|---|---|---|---|---|
| **SNACK** | | | | | | |
| | | | | | | |

NOTES:

| | FOOD | CAL. | | | | H$_2$O |
|---|---|---|---|---|---|---|
| **DINNER** | | | | | | |
| | | | | | | |
| | | | | | | |

NOTES:

| | | | | | | |
|---|---|---|---|---|---|---|
| **SNACK** | | | | | | |

NOTES:

| EXERCISE TYPE | 15 MIN. | 30 MIN. | 45 MIN. | 60 MIN. |
|---|---|---|---|---|
| | | | | |

# SUNDAY

| | FOOD | CAL. | | | | H₂O |
|---|---|---|---|---|---|---|
| **BREAKFAST** | | | | | | |
| | | | | | | |
| | | | | | | |
| | | | | | | |

NOTES:

| | FOOD | CAL. | | | | H₂O |
|---|---|---|---|---|---|---|
| **SNACK** | | | | | | |
| | | | | | | |

NOTES:

| | FOOD | CAL. | | | | H₂O |
|---|---|---|---|---|---|---|
| **LUNCH** | | | | | | |
| | | | | | | |
| | | | | | | |
| | | | | | | |

NOTES:

| | FOOD | CAL. | | | | H₂O |
|---|---|---|---|---|---|---|
| **SNACK** | | | | | | |
| | | | | | | |

NOTES:

| | FOOD | CAL. | | | | H₂O |
|---|---|---|---|---|---|---|
| **DINNER** | | | | | | |
| | | | | | | |
| | | | | | | |
| | | | | | | |

NOTES:

| **SNACK** | | | | | |
|---|---|---|---|---|---|

NOTES:

| EXERCISE TYPE | 15 MIN. | 30 MIN. | 45 MIN. | 60 MIN. |
|---|---|---|---|---|
| | | | | |

# The *Bite It and Write It* Shopping List

Our shopping guide is meant to be a reusable tool. Photocopy the list below and consult it each week when planning your meals and supermarket trips. We have focused on healthy foods that we feel are the most vital for maintaining a nutritious diet. Along with an extensive list of groceries, we have included some of our favorite food brands to make shopping less confusing and overwhelming.

## WHOLE GRAIN CEREALS

### Cold Cereals

- ☐ All-Bran
- ☐ Barbara's Bakery Puffins, original or cinnamon
- ☐ Barbara's Bakery Shredded Spoonfuls
- ☐ Barbara's Bakery Ultima Organic Slim
- ☐ Bare Naked Granola
- ☐ Cascadian Farm Hearty Morning Fiber
- ☐ Cheerios
- ☐ Kashi GOLEAN
- ☐ Kashi Heart to Heart
- ☐ Kashi 7 Whole Grain Flakes
- ☐ Nature's Path Smart Bran
- ☐ Nature's Path Organic Optimum
- ☐ Simply Fiber
- ☐ Special K Protein Plus

### Hot Cereals

- ☐ Hodgson Mill Multi Grain Hot Cereal
- ☐ Hodgson Mill Oat Bran Hot Cereal (any brand is acceptable)
- ☐ Kashi GOLEAN Hot Cereal,
- Hearty Honey Cinnamon Oatmeal
- ☐ Kashi GOLEAN Hot Cereal, Creamy Truly Vanilla
- ☐ Nature's Path Organic Hot
- Oatmeal
- ☐ McCann's Irish Oatmeal
- ☐ Quaker High Fiber Instant Oatmeal
- ☐ Steel cut oats

## FRUITS

- ❑ Apples
- ❑ Apricots
- ❑ Avocados
- ❑ Bananas
- ❑ Berries (blackberries, blueberries, raspberries, strawberries, Cascadian Farm frozen berries)
- ❑ Cherries
- ❑ Figs
- ❑ Grapefruit
- ❑ Grapes
- ❑ Guava
- ❑ Kiwi
- ❑ Lemon
- ❑ Limes
- ❑ Mangos
- ❑ Melon (cantaloupe, honeydew, watermelon)
- ❑ Nectarines
- ❑ Oranges (navel, clementines)
- ❑ Papaya
- ❑ Peaches
- ❑ Pears
- ❑ Pineapple
- ❑ Plums
- ❑ Pomegranates
- ❑ Tangerines

## VEGETABLES

- ❑ Artichokes
- ❑ Beets
- ❑ Bok choy
- ❑ Broccoli
- ❑ Brussels sprouts
- ❑ Cabbage (red and/or white)
- ❑ Carrots
- ❑ Cauliflower
- ❑ Celery
- ❑ Cucumbers
- ❑ Eggplant
- ❑ Fennel
- ❑ Green beans
- ❑ Jicama
- ❑ Kale
- ❑ Leeks
- ❑ Mushrooms
- ❑ Onions
- ❑ Peppers (green, orange, red, jalapeño)
- ❑ Radishes
- ❑ Salad greens
- ❑ Scallions
- ❑ Snow peas
- ❑ Spinach
- ❑ Tomatoes
- ❑ Watercress
- ❑ Zucchini

### Starchy Vegetables

- ❑ Acorn squash
- ❑ Butternut squash
- ❑ Corn
- ❑ Potatoes (white, red)
- ❑ Sweet potatoes

### Frozen Vegetables

- ❑ Birds Eye Fresh
- ❑ Green Giant Steamers

## DAIRY

- ❑ Cheese
  - • low-fat 2% Cabot Cheddar
  - • Kraft Deli Fresh Swiss
  - • Laughing Cow, light varieties
- • Farmer's cheese
- ❑ Cottage cheese, low-sodium brands (Friendship, 1% milk fat)
- ❑ Milk
  - • low-fat or fat-free
- ❑ Yogurt (organic and under 150 calories)
  - • Dannon Naturals
  - • Stonyfield Farm, plain or flavors
  - • Greek, low-fat, plain or flavors

## BREADS AND GRAINS

*Buy bread products that are no more than 100 calories per serving and contain at least 3 grams of fiber per serving.*

- ❑ Barley
- ❑ Black and/or brown rice
- ❑ Bulgar
- ❑ Quinoa
- ❑ 100% whole wheat bread, rye bread, or other whole grain bread (Matthew's All Natural, Pepperidge Farm,
Trader Joe's, Vermont Bakery)
- ❑ 100% whole wheat English muffins (Fiber One, Matthew's All Natural, Trader Joe's)
- ❑ 100% whole wheat mini bagels (Thomas)
- ❑ 100% whole wheat pita (Pepperidge Farm mini, Trader Joe's, and Sahara)
- ❑ 100% whole wheat wraps (La Tortilla Factory, Damascus Bakeries)

## NUTS, LEGUMES, AND BEANS (canned or dry)

- ❑ Black beans
- ❑ Cannellini beans
- ❑ Chickpeas (Gabanzo beans)
- ❑ Edamame
- ❑ Kidney beans
- ❑ Lentils
- ❑ Nuts (almonds, cashews, hazel-
nuts, walnuts, etc.)
- ❑ Split peas
- ❑ Vegetarian refried beans, fat-free

## SWEETENERS

- ❑ Agave nectar
- ❑ Honey
- ❑ Organic sugar

## LEAN PROTEIN

- Beef, lean cuts only: bottom round, eye round, sirloin tip, top round, top sirloin
- Eggs/Egg whites
- Fish/Shellfish
  - Bronzini
  - Cod
  - Halibut
- Lobster
- Salmon, organic or wild (fresh or canned)
- Sardines
- Scallops
- Sea bass
- Shrimp
- Sole
- Tuna, light (canned in water)
- Ham (fresh)
- Pork, tenderloin or center loin
- Poultry breast, skinless
- Processed deli meats, Applegate Farms brand only (does not contain nitrates)

## PREPARED FOODS

### Entrées and Sides

- Amy's Kitchen
- Garden Lites

### Vegetarian Options

- BOCA Veggie Burgers
- Dr. Praeger's California Veggie Burgers
- Dr. Praeger's Spinach Pancakes
- Morningstar Farms Veggie Burgers
- Seaweed Noodles (Kombu)
- Tempeh (Lightlife Organic)
- Tofu (Mori Nu, Nayosa)

### Soups, low sodium

- Select Harvest
- Progresso, Light brand (0 points)
- Health Valley

## FATS AND OILS

- Butter, whipped (light or Smart Balance spread, all varieties)
- Nut butters (almond, cashew, sunflower seed, all natural peanut butter)
- Oils (coconut, olive, safflower, sesame)

## SNACK FOODS

- Crackers
  - FiberRich bran crackers
  - Finn Crisp
  - GG Scandinavian Crispbread
  - Wasa
- Desserts
  - Glenny's brownies or cookies
  - Skinny Cow frozen desserts
- Dips
  - Black bean dip (Guiltless Gourmet)
  - Guacamole (Trader Joe's or Wholly Guacamole)
  - Hummus (Cedar's, Sabra, Trader Joe's, or Tribe brands)
- Fruit
  - Cubed coconut
  - Dried fruit (Just Apples brand)
- Muffins
  - Muffin Delite Supremes
  - Vitalicious VitaMuffins or VitaTops
- Nuts (Blue Diamond 100-calorie packs)
- Popcorn, fresh kernels for air-popping, or:
  - Bachman Light
  - Boston Lite
  - Jolly Time 100-calorie microwave popcorn
  - Newman's Own, Light Butter
  - Orville Redenbacher Mini Bags (94% Fat-Free)
  - Smart Balance Light Butter
- Snack bars (Clif, Gnu, KIND, LUNA)

## CONDIMENTS

- Horseradish (white)
- Hot sauce
- Ketchup (Heinz Reduced Sugar/No Salt Added, Muir Glen Organic)
- Marinara sauce (Amy's, Mamma Lombardi's, Colavita Organic)
- Mayonnaise (Hellman's Low-Fat, Spectrum brand)
- Mustard
- Pesto
- Salad dressings, light varieties (no more than 75 calories per every 2 tablespoons; Annie's Naturals)
- Salsa
- Soy sauce (low sodium)
- Vinegars, 0-calorie (apple cider, balsamic, brown rice, red wine)

# Goal 4

## Eat Breakfast Each Day, and You'll Like What You Weigh

I t is a common misconception that the less you eat, the quicker you lose weight. Though far from the truth, this mistaken belief often causes dieters to skip meals, and breakfast is usually the first to go. The rationale usually goes something like this: "I'm not that hungry in the morning, so isn't it better if I save my calories for later in the day?" The answer to this question, very simply, is *no*. In the same way that a car needs gas to start its engine, the human body needs food in order to properly function and maintain sufficient energy levels. Breakfast is the meal that jumpstarts your metabolism each day and gives you a much-needed energy boost in the morning. As researchers have consistently found, the more regularly you eat breakfast, the less you will probably weigh.

Our clients give similar reasons for skipping breakfast. One of the more common ones is the always-popular "Breakfast makes me hungrier" excuse. Though hunger is a sign of a healthy and efficient metabolism, many fear that a surge in appetite will lead to overeating at meals and consuming too many calories throughout the day. Breakfast is often viewed as the meal that opens the floodgates for eating, when, in actuality, it is the one that starts your body's metabolic cycle. A healthy, balanced breakfast with enough fiber and protein will keep you satisfied until your next meal or snack, not set in motion a streak of overindulging.

Another common excuse for skipping breakfast is not having enough time in the morning. While we certainly understand how busy schedules can interfere with your ability to enjoy a relaxed meal, omitting the most important meal of the day is never acceptable. Breakfast needs to become an integral part of your morning routine just like brushing your teeth and getting dressed. If you cannot sit down and eat (which would be preferable), then grab something (healthy!) that you can eat during your commute.

The consequences of skipping breakfast are adverse to your nutrition, weight loss success, and overall health. When you do not eat in the morning, your blood sugar levels plummet, which triggers cravings for simple sugars that are empty in nutrients and high in calories. Low blood sugar levels will also cause you to make poor food choices, or worse, overeat. This is especially true when you also miss lunch, since skipping two essential meals will cause a further slump in blood sugar followed by binging at dinner and probable mood swings. You should never feel "starved" or extremely hungry, as this indicates that you have allowed your hunger to spiral out of control—a surefire way *not* to meet your nutritional goals.

Simply put, your goal is to eat three meals a day—breakfast, lunch, and dinner—no more than four to six hours apart. If you are unable to eat meals every few hours, a sensible "mini meal" or snack can help to alleviate hunger and bridge longer gaps between mealtimes. Eating at regular intervals is advantageous to your physical and mental well-being: You boost your metabolism, temper mood swings, and feel more energetic.

Break your meal-skipping habits by following our advice:

☑ **Eat breakfast daily.** As we explained, breakfast is the meal that fuels your body's system and jumpstarts its metabolism, so start your day mindfully by eating a nutritious and balanced breakfast of high-fiber carbohydrates, protein, and/or low-fat dairy. Current research finds that incorporating a source of healthy fat into your breakfast such as eggs, avocado, or nuts will give your metabolism an even bigger boost. In other words, eating breakfast sets your day up for success.

☑ **Plan your meals and snacks every day.** If you always know what you will eat next, you'll never find yourself making poor food choices due to hunger, cravings, or mood swings. For example, if you buy a sandwich at the local deli for lunch, also grab a serving of fruit or yogurt for your afternoon snack. Always think one step ahead and anticipate when you will be ready to eat again—planning is the key to success!

☑ **Always have a sensible snack on hand.** Keeping healthy snack bars or small pre-packaged bags of nuts in your car during the day will keep your hunger levels at bay and prevent you from skipping meals. Refer to our chart on pages 98 to 100 for a list of healthy snacks that are both satisfying and low in calories.

☑ **Never be "too busy" to eat.** In order to accomplish your nutrition and weight loss goals, you need to make yourself a priority. *You* are important. *You* deserve to be healthy. Therefore, *you* need to make time for meals and snacks. They do not need to be five-course meals at a fancy restaurant; just set aside a few moments each day to sit down, unwind, and eat.

By writing down the foods you eat, paying attention to portion size, and planning your trips to the supermarket, you have become a mindful eater. Going forward this week, you will focus on becoming a *timely* eater as well. You should look forward to your three meals each day, and eating a balanced breakfast along with certain "powerhouse" foods (see pages 72 to 74) will prevent you from going hungry or overeating. It takes effort to form healthy habits, but, over time, eating three meals a day—with sensible snacks in between—will become a natural part of your routine and an enjoyable part of your day.

Remember, in the process of achieving these smaller goals, you are developing the healthy eating habits necessary to change your lifestyle as well as your body, inside and out.

### WEEKLY PERSONAL GOAL

_____

_____

_____

_____

### WEEKLY CONCLUSION

_____

_____

_____

_____

# MONDAY

| | FOOD | CAL. | | | | H₂O |
|---|---|---|---|---|---|---|
| **BREAKFAST** | | | | | | 🥤 |
| | | | | | | 🥤 |
| | | | | | | 🥤 |
| | | | | | | |

NOTES:

| | | | | | | H₂O |
|---|---|---|---|---|---|---|
| **SNACK** | | | | | | 🥤 |
| | | | | | | 🥤 |

NOTES:

| | | | | | | H₂O |
|---|---|---|---|---|---|---|
| **LUNCH** | | | | | | 🥤 |
| | | | | | | 🥤 |
| | | | | | | 🥤 |
| | | | | | | |

NOTES:

| | | | | | | H₂O |
|---|---|---|---|---|---|---|
| **SNACK** | | | | | | 🥤 |
| | | | | | | 🥤 |

NOTES:

| | | | | | | H₂O |
|---|---|---|---|---|---|---|
| **DINNER** | | | | | | 🥤 |
| | | | | | | 🥤 |
| | | | | | | 🥤 |
| | | | | | | |

NOTES:

| **SNACK** | | | | | 🥤 |
|---|---|---|---|---|---|

NOTES:

| EXERCISE TYPE | 15 MIN. | 30 MIN. | 45 MIN. | 60 MIN. |
|---|---|---|---|---|
| | | | | |

# TUESDAY

| | FOOD | CAL. | | | | H₂O |
|---|---|---|---|---|---|---|
| **BREAKFAST** | | | | | | |
| | | | | | | |
| | | | | | | |
| | | | | | | |

NOTES: _____

| | | | | | | H₂O |
|---|---|---|---|---|---|---|
| **SNACK** | | | | | | |
| | | | | | | |

NOTES: _____

| | | | | | | H₂O |
|---|---|---|---|---|---|---|
| **LUNCH** | | | | | | |
| | | | | | | |
| | | | | | | |
| | | | | | | |

NOTES: _____

| | | | | | | H₂O |
|---|---|---|---|---|---|---|
| **SNACK** | | | | | | |
| | | | | | | |

NOTES: _____

| | | | | | | H₂O |
|---|---|---|---|---|---|---|
| **DINNER** | | | | | | |
| | | | | | | |
| | | | | | | |

NOTES: _____

| | | | | | | |
|---|---|---|---|---|---|---|
| **SNACK** | | | | | | |

NOTES:

| EXERCISE TYPE | 15 MIN. | 30 MIN. | 45 MIN. | 60 MIN. |
|---|---|---|---|---|
| | | | | |

| WEDNESDAY | FOOD | CAL. | | | | H₂O |
|-----------|------|------|---|---|---|-----|
| **BREAKFAST** | | | | | | 🥤 🥤 🥤 |

NOTES: _____

| **SNACK** | | | | | | 🥤 🥤 |

NOTES: _____

| **LUNCH** | | | | | | 🥤 🥤 🥤 |

NOTES: _____

| **SNACK** | | | | | | 🥤 🥤 |

NOTES: _____

| **DINNER** | | | | | | 🥤 🥤 🥤 |

NOTES: _____

| **SNACK** | | | | | | 🥤 |

NOTES: _____

| EXERCISE TYPE | 15 MIN. | 30 MIN. | 45 MIN. | 60 MIN. |
|---------------|---------|---------|---------|---------|
| | | | | |

# THURSDAY

| | FOOD | CAL. | | | | H₂O |
|---|---|---|---|---|---|---|
| **BREAKFAST** | | | | | | 🥤 |
| | | | | | | 🥤 |
| | | | | | | 🥤 |
| | | | | | | 🥤 |

NOTES: _____

| | FOOD | CAL. | | | | H₂O |
|---|---|---|---|---|---|---|
| **SNACK** | | | | | | 🥤 |
| | | | | | | 🥤 |

NOTES: _____

| | FOOD | CAL. | | | | H₂O |
|---|---|---|---|---|---|---|
| **LUNCH** | | | | | | 🥤 |
| | | | | | | 🥤 |
| | | | | | | 🥤 |
| | | | | | | 🥤 |

NOTES: _____

| | FOOD | CAL. | | | | H₂O |
|---|---|---|---|---|---|---|
| **SNACK** | | | | | | 🥤 |
| | | | | | | 🥤 |

NOTES: _____

| | FOOD | CAL. | | | | H₂O |
|---|---|---|---|---|---|---|
| **DINNER** | | | | | | 🥤 |
| | | | | | | 🥤 |
| | | | | | | 🥤 |
| | | | | | | 🥤 |

NOTES: _____

| | | | | | | H₂O |
|---|---|---|---|---|---|---|
| **SNACK** | | | | | | 🥤 |

NOTES: _____

| EXERCISE TYPE | 15 MIN. | 30 MIN. | 45 MIN. | 60 MIN. |
|---|---|---|---|---|
| | | | | |

| FRIDAY | FOOD | CAL. | | | | H₂O |
|---|---|---|---|---|---|---|
| **BREAKFAST** | | | | | | 🥤 |
| | | | | | | 🥤 |
| | | | | | | 🥤 |
| | | | | | | |

NOTES: _____

| **SNACK** | | | | | | 🥤 |
|---|---|---|---|---|---|---|
| | | | | | | 🥤 |

NOTES: _____

| **LUNCH** | | | | | | 🥤 |
|---|---|---|---|---|---|---|
| | | | | | | 🥤 |
| | | | | | | 🥤 |
| | | | | | | |

NOTES: _____

| **SNACK** | | | | | | 🥤 |
|---|---|---|---|---|---|---|
| | | | | | | 🥤 |

NOTES: _____

| **DINNER** | | | | | | 🥤 |
|---|---|---|---|---|---|---|
| | | | | | | 🥤 |
| | | | | | | 🥤 |
| | | | | | | |

NOTES: _____

| **SNACK** | | | | | | 🥤 |
|---|---|---|---|---|---|---|

NOTES: _____

| EXERCISE TYPE | 15 MIN. | 30 MIN. | 45 MIN. | 60 MIN. |
|---|---|---|---|---|
| | | | | |

# SATURDAY

| | FOOD | CAL. | | | | H$_2$O |
|---|---|---|---|---|---|---|
| **BREAKFAST** | | | | | | 🥤 |
| | | | | | | 🥤 |
| | | | | | | 🥤 |
| | | | | | | |

NOTES: _____

| | FOOD | CAL. | | | | H$_2$O |
|---|---|---|---|---|---|---|
| **SNACK** | | | | | | 🥤 |
| | | | | | | 🥤 |

NOTES: _____

| | FOOD | CAL. | | | | H$_2$O |
|---|---|---|---|---|---|---|
| **LUNCH** | | | | | | 🥤 |
| | | | | | | 🥤 |
| | | | | | | 🥤 |
| | | | | | | |

NOTES: _____

| | FOOD | CAL. | | | | H$_2$O |
|---|---|---|---|---|---|---|
| **SNACK** | | | | | | 🥤 |
| | | | | | | 🥤 |

NOTES: _____

| | FOOD | CAL. | | | | H$_2$O |
|---|---|---|---|---|---|---|
| **DINNER** | | | | | | 🥤 |
| | | | | | | 🥤 |
| | | | | | | 🥤 |
| | | | | | | |

NOTES: _____

| | FOOD | CAL. | | | | H$_2$O |
|---|---|---|---|---|---|---|
| **SNACK** | | | | | | 🥤 |

NOTES: _____

| EXERCISE TYPE | 15 MIN. | 30 MIN. | 45 MIN. | 60 MIN. |
|---|---|---|---|---|
| | | | | |

# SUNDAY

| | FOOD | CAL. | | | | H₂O |
|---|---|---|---|---|---|---|
| **BREAKFAST** | | | | | | |
| | | | | | | |
| | | | | | | |
| | | | | | | |

NOTES:

| | FOOD | CAL. | | | | H₂O |
|---|---|---|---|---|---|---|
| **SNACK** | | | | | | |
| | | | | | | |

NOTES:

| | FOOD | CAL. | | | | H₂O |
|---|---|---|---|---|---|---|
| **LUNCH** | | | | | | |
| | | | | | | |
| | | | | | | |
| | | | | | | |

NOTES:

| | FOOD | CAL. | | | | H₂O |
|---|---|---|---|---|---|---|
| **SNACK** | | | | | | |
| | | | | | | |

NOTES:

| | FOOD | CAL. | | | | H₂O |
|---|---|---|---|---|---|---|
| **DINNER** | | | | | | |
| | | | | | | |
| | | | | | | |
| | | | | | | |

NOTES:

| | | | | | | |
|---|---|---|---|---|---|---|
| **SNACK** | | | | | | |

NOTES:

| EXERCISE TYPE | 15 MIN. | 30 MIN. | 45 MIN. | 60 MIN. |
|---|---|---|---|---|
| | | | | |

# Top Ten "Super" Foods

While we love several healthy foods, there are a select few that we constantly recommend to our clients. Based on sound research, the choices listed below are our top ten nutritional powerhouse foods, and we urge you to include them in your diet as you continue your weight loss journey. So, let's cut to the chase and give you the juice!

**1. Almonds.** Yes, it's true: There are foods that can be high in fat and also good for your health, and almonds are one such food. They contain "healthy fat" that is not only good for your heart, but also for your waistline. Dietary fat is not converted into body fat when it is consumed in modest amounts, so enjoy 1 ounce of almonds (about 15) each day.

**2. Blueberries.** These berries are a true blue food, but there's no need to be sad! The "blue" in a blueberry is actually a powerful antioxidant called anthocyanin, which makes it one of the most antioxidant-rich foods. In addition, blueberries are a great source of fiber and vitamin C, so eating them is a perfect way to satisfy your craving for something sweet.

**Tip:** You can get your blueberries to ripen more quickly by placing them in a bag with an apple. Apples contain the hormone ethylene, which promotes the ripening of fruit.

**3. Asparagus.** If you feel bloated, enjoy the diuretic benefits of this vegetable. Even better, asparagus contains a high amount of glutathione, which is one of the body's most potent cancer fighters. A member of the lily family, asparagus is notoriously known for its strong, distinct odor. But do not be alarmed by this pungent smell: It's merely a signal that your body has absorbed the vegetable's nutrients and is using them.

**Tip:** In the supermarket, look for firm asparagus that has a rich green color, tightly closed heads, and freshly cut ends. It is best to eat asparagus soon after it has been purchased.

**4. Salmon.** Salmon contains high amounts of EPA and DHA, which are omega-3 fatty acids essential for disease prevention. Omega-3 fatty acids also protect arteries, improve mental health, sharpen vision, and bolster your immunity.

**Tip:** Always buy wild caught salmon. It contains the most omega-3 fatty acids and none of the chemicals found in farm raised salmon. Due to its mercury content, pregnant and nursing women should limit their intake to 12 ounces a week.

**5. Yogurt.** After being introduced in the United States, yogurt was initially sold in pharmacies and considered to have medicinal properties. Yogurt has many gastrointestinal benefits because it is abundant in probiotics, "pacman"-like microorganisms that absorb harmful bacteria in the stomach and fortify the body's immune system. In addition, yogurt is an excellent source of calcium, which protects your bones and strengthens your heart.

**6. Lentils.** Do not be deceived by size: These tiny legumes are packed with benefits. Lentils contain twice as much iron as other legumes, not to mention antioxidants, protein, and soluble fiber that can lower cholesterol. Moreover, lentils are high in other vital nutrients like B vitamins and folate, so this little bean will take you a long way.

**7. Sweet Potatoes.** Loaded with beta-carotene and fiber, sweet potatoes are as healthy as they are delicious. Since they are already portion-controlled for you (prepackaged in their own skin) and high in fiber, they make the perfect carbohydrate accompaniment to your dinner.

**Tip:** When buying sweet potatoes, make sure they are heavy (for their size), firm, and have a tight skin. Also be sure that they do not have any unsightly spots, sprouts, or mold.

**8. Avocados.** There are two things that may surprise you about avocados. First, they are actually a fruit, not a vegetable. Second, they contain a considerable amount of monounsaturated fat, which promotes a healthy heart. When eaten in moderation, avocados have numerous benefits: They can lower cholesterol, decrease your risk of heart disease, and help you to feel fuller after a meal by slowing your digestive process.

**Tip:** There are many varieties of avocados (each with its own "season"), so they can be bought at your local supermarket year round. It's best to buy them when they are still slightly green and firm, and then let them ripen in your home. Ripe avocados can be stored in your refrigerator for up to a week.

**9. Tea.** Drink to your health! Tea of all kinds—green, black, white, and herbal—contain compounds that guard against life-threatening diseases such as cancer and heart disease. So sit back, relax, and enjoy a cup of your favorite tea, along with all the benefits that come with it.

**10. Eggs.** When it comes to nutrition, there's no such thing as a bad egg. Eggs are loaded with choline, a compound that improves cognitive development and function; eating just one will boost brainwaves and sharpen your memory. Eggs (especially the yolks) are also an excellent source of protein, so making them a part of your breakfast will satisfy your appetite and cause you to eat less throughout the day, which also means you will *weigh* less. Just remember to keep your consumption of egg yolks to no more than four or five a week.

# Goal 5

## Keep Drinking— Water, That Is

Drinking water is vital to your health, yet you are probably not drinking as much as your body requires. Few people meet their daily water requirements, and most overlook the positive effects that water can have on their nutritional well-being. In addition to controlling your weight, drinking water regularly will prevent dehydration, boost your metabolism, enhance bowel regularity, relieve bloating and swelling, and improve the appearance of your skin. When it comes to quenching your thirst, water is always the way to go.

How much water is enough? Though precise amounts vary by weight (refer to the chart on page 76), on average, a person should drink eight 8-ounce glasses of water each day. This may seem excessive or difficult to work into your schedule, but drinking eight glasses of water daily is as essential as eating three meals a day. We recommend drinking a 16-ounce glass of water in the morning, an additional 16 ounces between each meal, and your last two glasses after dinner. Drinking water at regular intervals will consistently hydrate your body.

You will probably notice that increasing your daily water intake results in more frequent urination. This has its perks: Urinating allows you to remove toxins from your body, move your bowels easier, and avoid excessive gas.

Urine that is lighter in color is an indication of healthiness and hydration, so you'll always know whether or not you're drinking enough water.

It is also important to bear in mind that thirst is often mistaken for hunger. When you are not properly hydrated, your body sends signals to your brain that may cause you to think you're hungry. All you may need is a glass of water— so remember this, and drink up before you snack away.

Here are five ways you can make water a basic part of your day:

**1. Begin your day with a 16-ounce glass of water.** You always wake up dehydrated, so start your day the right way by rehydrating. Drinking water before or with breakfast will make you feel fuller and less inclined to snack during the mid-morning hours. Adding freshly squeezed lemon juice to your morning glass will also help to detoxify and balance your body's system.

**2. Travel with a water bottle.** Carry a 32-ounce water bottle with you (to work, to school, or when you run errands), and

## Your Daily Water Requirements

| | RECOMMENDED WATER INTAKE | |
|---|---|---|
| BODY WEIGHT | IN OUNCES | IN CUPS |
| 100-120 lbs | 48 | 6 |
| 121-140 lbs | 48-64 | 6-8 |
| 141-160 lbs | 56-72 | 7-9 |
| 161-180 lbs | 64-80 | 8-10 |
| 181-200 lbs | 72-88 | 9-11 |
| Greater than 225 | Greater than 90 | Greater than 12 |

try to finish it over the course of the day. This will leave you with only two more glasses of water to drink for the day. Consuming these two remaining glasses of water after dinner will allow the food in your stomach to expand, which keeps you feeling full. Try using a stainless steel water bottle to keep your water cold and prevent plastic from leaching into your water on hot days.

**3. Drink water with meals.** Substituting water for soda, juice, and alcohol saves you tons of calories, not to mention money. Water is the best way to hydrate your body.

**4. Drink water before eating a snack.** Sometimes all it takes is a glass of water to keep you satisfied. Drinking water will allow you to determine whether you're hungry or simply thirsty. If food is truly what you need, washing down your healthy snack with a glass of water will aid the digestive process.

**5. Stop buying soda.** If you buy it, you will drink it. Eliminate the temptation altogether and leave yourself with no choice but a refreshing glass of water.

There is no excuse *not* to drink water. Fit in your eight glasses each day, and you will notice vast improvements. If you're bored with the taste (or lack thereof), a small amount of freshly squeezed lemon juice will add some flavor. Once you get in the habit of drinking water, it will become an accepted part of your routine. All you have to do is start.

Aside from serving as an essential element in your nutritional well-being, water is also necessary for physical fitness. Water loosens your joints, protects muscle tissue, and prevents dehydration, which will allow your body to perform at its best during exercise. Generally, you should aim to drink 2 ounces of water per every 15 minutes of exercise, which is in addition to your basic daily requirement. Daily requirements largely depend upon weight but increase with the heat index. If the temperature outside is above 75 degrees, you should consume an extra 8 ounces of water for every hour you spend outdoors. Use the chart on page 76 to determine your basic daily requirement, and adjust it according to both the temperature and duration of physical activity.

## WEEKLY PERSONAL GOAL

_____

_____

_____

_____

_____

_____

## WEEKLY CONCLUSION

_____

_____

_____

_____

_____

_____

_____

# MONDAY

| | FOOD | CAL. | | | | H₂O |
|---|---|---|---|---|---|---|
| **BREAKFAST** | | | | | | 🥤 |
| | | | | | | 🥤 |
| | | | | | | 🥤 |
| | | | | | | |

NOTES: _____

| | | | | | | H₂O |
|---|---|---|---|---|---|---|
| **SNACK** | | | | | | 🥤 |
| | | | | | | 🥤 |

NOTES: _____

| | | | | | | H₂O |
|---|---|---|---|---|---|---|
| **LUNCH** | | | | | | 🥤 |
| | | | | | | 🥤 |
| | | | | | | 🥤 |

NOTES: _____

| | | | | | | H₂O |
|---|---|---|---|---|---|---|
| **SNACK** | | | | | | 🥤 |
| | | | | | | 🥤 |

NOTES: _____

| | | | | | | H₂O |
|---|---|---|---|---|---|---|
| **DINNER** | | | | | | 🥤 |
| | | | | | | 🥤 |
| | | | | | | 🥤 |

NOTES: _____

| **SNACK** | | | | | | 🥤 |
|---|---|---|---|---|---|---|

NOTES: _____

| EXERCISE TYPE | 15 MIN. | 30 MIN. | 45 MIN. | 60 MIN. |
|---|---|---|---|---|
| | | | | |

| TUESDAY | FOOD | CAL. | | | | H₂O |
|---|---|---|---|---|---|---|
| **BREAKFAST** | | | | | | 🥤 |
| | | | | | | 🥤 |
| | | | | | | 🥤 |
| | | | | | | |

NOTES: _____

| **SNACK** | | | | | | 🥤 |
|---|---|---|---|---|---|---|
| | | | | | | 🥤 |

NOTES: _____

| **LUNCH** | | | | | | 🥤 |
|---|---|---|---|---|---|---|
| | | | | | | 🥤 |
| | | | | | | 🥤 |
| | | | | | | |

NOTES: _____

| **SNACK** | | | | | | 🥤 |
|---|---|---|---|---|---|---|
| | | | | | | 🥤 |

NOTES: _____

| **DINNER** | | | | | | 🥤 |
|---|---|---|---|---|---|---|
| | | | | | | 🥤 |
| | | | | | | 🥤 |
| | | | | | | |

NOTES: _____

| **SNACK** | | | | | 🥤 |
|---|---|---|---|---|---|

NOTES: _____

| EXERCISE TYPE | 15 MIN. | 30 MIN. | 45 MIN. | 60 MIN. |
|---|---|---|---|---|
| | | | | |

## WEDNESDAY

| BREAKFAST | FOOD | CAL. | | | | H₂O |
|---|---|---|---|---|---|---|
| | | | | | | 🥤 |
| | | | | | | 🥤 |
| | | | | | | 🥤 |

NOTES:

| SNACK | | | | | | H₂O |
|---|---|---|---|---|---|---|
| | | | | | | 🥤 |
| | | | | | | 🥤 |

NOTES:

| LUNCH | | | | | | |
|---|---|---|---|---|---|---|
| | | | | | | 🥤 |
| | | | | | | 🥤 |
| | | | | | | 🥤 |

NOTES:

| SNACK | | | | | | |
|---|---|---|---|---|---|---|
| | | | | | | 🥤 |
| | | | | | | 🥤 |

NOTES:

| DINNER | | | | | | |
|---|---|---|---|---|---|---|
| | | | | | | 🥤 |
| | | | | | | 🥤 |
| | | | | | | 🥤 |

NOTES:

| SNACK | | | | | | 🥤 |
|---|---|---|---|---|---|---|

NOTES:

| EXERCISE TYPE | 15 MIN. | 30 MIN. | 45 MIN. | 60 MIN. |
|---|---|---|---|---|
| | | | | |

# THURSDAY

| | FOOD | CAL. | | | | H₂O |
|---|---|---|---|---|---|---|
| **BREAKFAST** | | | | | | 🥤 |
| | | | | | | 🥤 |
| | | | | | | 🥤 |
| | | | | | | |

NOTES: _____

| | FOOD | CAL. | | | | H₂O |
|---|---|---|---|---|---|---|
| **SNACK** | | | | | | 🥤 |
| | | | | | | 🥤 |

NOTES: _____

| | FOOD | CAL. | | | | H₂O |
|---|---|---|---|---|---|---|
| **LUNCH** | | | | | | 🥤 |
| | | | | | | 🥤 |
| | | | | | | 🥤 |
| | | | | | | |

NOTES: _____

| | FOOD | CAL. | | | | H₂O |
|---|---|---|---|---|---|---|
| **SNACK** | | | | | | 🥤 |
| | | | | | | 🥤 |

NOTES: _____

| | FOOD | CAL. | | | | H₂O |
|---|---|---|---|---|---|---|
| **DINNER** | | | | | | 🥤 |
| | | | | | | 🥤 |
| | | | | | | 🥤 |
| | | | | | | |

NOTES: _____

| | | | | | | |
|---|---|---|---|---|---|---|
| **SNACK** | | | | | | 🥤 |

NOTES: _____

| EXERCISE TYPE | 15 MIN. | 30 MIN. | 45 MIN. | 60 MIN. |
|---|---|---|---|---|
| | | | | |

## FRIDAY

| | FOOD | CAL. | | | | H₂O |
|---|---|---|---|---|---|---|
| **BREAKFAST** | | | | | | 🥤 |
| | | | | | | 🥤 |
| | | | | | | 🥤 |
| | | | | | | |

NOTES: _____

| | | | | | | H₂O |
|---|---|---|---|---|---|---|
| **SNACK** | | | | | | 🥤 |
| | | | | | | 🥤 |

NOTES: _____

| | | | | | | H₂O |
|---|---|---|---|---|---|---|
| **LUNCH** | | | | | | 🥤 |
| | | | | | | 🥤 |
| | | | | | | 🥤 |
| | | | | | | |

NOTES: _____

| | | | | | | H₂O |
|---|---|---|---|---|---|---|
| **SNACK** | | | | | | 🥤 |
| | | | | | | 🥤 |

NOTES: _____

| | | | | | | H₂O |
|---|---|---|---|---|---|---|
| **DINNER** | | | | | | 🥤 |
| | | | | | | 🥤 |
| | | | | | | 🥤 |
| | | | | | | |

NOTES: _____

| **SNACK** | | | | | | 🥤 |
|---|---|---|---|---|---|---|

NOTES: _____

| EXERCISE TYPE | 15 MIN. | 30 MIN. | 45 MIN. | 60 MIN. |
|---|---|---|---|---|
| | | | | |

## SATURDAY

| | FOOD | CAL. | | | | H₂O |
|---|---|---|---|---|---|---|
| **BREAKFAST** | | | | | | 🥛 |
| | | | | | | 🥛 |
| | | | | | | 🥛 |
| | | | | | | |

NOTES: _____

| | FOOD | CAL. | | | | H₂O |
|---|---|---|---|---|---|---|
| **SNACK** | | | | | | 🥛 |
| | | | | | | 🥛 |

NOTES: _____

| | FOOD | CAL. | | | | H₂O |
|---|---|---|---|---|---|---|
| **LUNCH** | | | | | | 🥛 |
| | | | | | | 🥛 |
| | | | | | | 🥛 |

NOTES: _____

| | FOOD | CAL. | | | | H₂O |
|---|---|---|---|---|---|---|
| **SNACK** | | | | | | 🥛 |
| | | | | | | 🥛 |

NOTES: _____

| | FOOD | CAL. | | | | H₂O |
|---|---|---|---|---|---|---|
| **DINNER** | | | | | | 🥛 |
| | | | | | | 🥛 |
| | | | | | | 🥛 |

NOTES: _____

| | FOOD | CAL. | | | | H₂O |
|---|---|---|---|---|---|---|
| **SNACK** | | | | | | 🥛 |

NOTES: _____

| EXERCISE TYPE | 15 MIN. | 30 MIN. | 45 MIN. | 60 MIN. |
|---|---|---|---|---|
| | | | | |

| SUNDAY | FOOD | CAL. | | | | $H_2O$ |
|---|---|---|---|---|---|---|
| **BREAKFAST** | | | | | | 🍵 |
| | | | | | | 🍵 |
| | | | | | | 🍵 |
| | | | | | | |

NOTES: _____

| **SNACK** | | | | | | 🍵 |
|---|---|---|---|---|---|---|
| | | | | | | 🍵 |

NOTES: _____

| **LUNCH** | | | | | | 🍵 |
|---|---|---|---|---|---|---|
| | | | | | | 🍵 |
| | | | | | | 🍵 |
| | | | | | | |

NOTES: _____

| **SNACK** | | | | | | 🍵 |
|---|---|---|---|---|---|---|
| | | | | | | 🍵 |

NOTES: _____

| **DINNER** | | | | | | 🍵 |
|---|---|---|---|---|---|---|
| | | | | | | 🍵 |
| | | | | | | 🍵 |
| | | | | | | |

NOTES: _____

| **SNACK** | | | | | | 🍵 |
|---|---|---|---|---|---|---|

NOTES: _____

| EXERCISE TYPE | 15 MIN. | 30 MIN. | 45 MIN. | 60 MIN. |
|---|---|---|---|---|
| | | | | |

# Go Green!

In this case, we're not talking about the environment. We're talking about what you should be drinking, if you aren't already: Green tea. Tea of any kind is a "nutritional powerhouse," but green tea in particular acts like a superhero in your body. Its disease-fighting properties, combined with its flavorful taste (it will grow on you, we promise), make green tea a healthy alternative to water.

Green tea is a natural "fighter" in your body, guarding against several types of cancer (breast, bladder, lung, colorectal, and prostate are a few), heart disease, and weight gain. Research has shown that nutrients found in green tea work to increase the rate at which you burn fat, and more remarkably, they target the fat in your belly. Drinking green tea will also balance your blood sugar and prevent the highs and lows that result in fatigue, irritability, and cravings for unhealthy food. Additional benefits include defense against skin damage and wrinkling. In other words, green tea keeps you healthy and youthful—and that's our kind of superhero!

The best way to reap the benefits of green tea is to drink it freshly brewed. Instant teas and decaffeinated ready-to-drink bottles have less potency, if any. Two to three cups a day is recommended, and there is no need to worry about caffeine—green tea contains less than coffee or black tea.

Follow our easy step-by-step directions below to brew yourself a mug of delicious green tea.

## How to Make Green Tea

1. Add one or two teaspoons of green tea leaves to a cup of boiling water, preferably in a tea strainer.

2. Let steep for three to five minutes.

3. Pour over ice if you prefer a cold beverage.

# Goal 6

## Snack Right, Be Light

**C**lients have often asked us, "What can I eat for a snack?" This question demonstrates that an effort is being made to eat mindfully by planning snacks and meals, so we encourage you to ask it. Our most successful clients are those who master the art of mindful snacking because it teaches you how to eat smaller portions, gauge your hunger and fullness levels, and be mentally in control of your eating. Planned snacks harness hunger, reduce the triggers that lead to binge eating, and help to stabilize your blood sugar.

The purpose of a snack is to provide energy and nutrients as well as sustain us between meals. Two planned snacks each day is usually sufficient. Ideally, your snacks should include some fruits and vegetables, as this allows you to meet two goals simultaneously: You will be eating mindfully and healthfully, and you will be increasing your daily intake from the two most important food groups (this will be discussed further in next week's goal, which begins on page 101). Nuts, whole grains, eggs, and low-fat cheeses are also great snack options. Keep in mind that there is a significant difference between a *snack* and a *treat*. Treats are foods that should only be eaten in limited quantities, such as cake, cookies, ice cream, and chips. Even when they are pre-portioned in 100-calorie bags, these foods contain nothing but empty calories. They are not nutritious, so they should not be staple snacks. If you find yourself craving foods like cookies and ice cream, stick to healthy brands and appropriate portions. Refer to our snack chart on pages 98 to 100 for further guidance in choosing snacks and treats that will satisfy your sweet (or salty) tooth.

You must also remember that "grazing" and "snacking" are two different things. Grazing generally indicates that your meals are not properly balanced or portioned, or that you are eating out of emotion rather than physical need. If you catch yourself grazing or wanting to eat more than your planned snacks and meals, you need to pay closer attention to what your body is telling you. Are you really hungry, or are you stressed, anxious, sad, or bored? This is where your food journal comes in: Write down why you wanted a snack and rank your level of hunger. If your desire to eat stems from emotions, consider how you can best address your feelings *without* food. Finding alternative solutions and remedies is probably the most difficult part of this process, but it can also be the most rewarding.

Here are some tips for becoming a master snacker:

• Shoot for snacks that are less than 200 calories. If your snack is packaged in larger bags or containers, measure out a serving that meets the recommended calorie range prior to eating. Our snack chart on pages 98 to 100 lists several suggestions for snacks that are both delicious and low in calories.

• Aim for nutritional balance. Snacks that contain protein, fiber-rich carbohydrates, and healthy fats will keep you satisfied longer and hold you over between meals. Hard-boiled eggs, nuts paired with a piece of fruit, and low-calorie soy crisps or veggie chips are sure to sustain you.

• Two snacks a day should be your limit. Either on your own or with your nutritionist, decide when it makes the most sense for you to have a snack based on when you are hungry and have available time. An afternoon snack is typically regarded as the most essential, since a longer gap of time falls between lunch and dinner than breakfast and lunch. Though most people prefer a snack in the evening rather than midmorning (when they are generally less hungry), midmorning snacks are important for those who exercise in the morning and need a boost of energy before lunch. Being a mindful eater, writing in your food journal regularly, and meeting with a nutritionist will help you identify the times during the day when a snack will be most beneficial for you.

• Be sure to eat a snack that contains carbohydrates and some protein after a workout that lasts for an hour or more. A piece of fruit, such as a small apple with 1 tablespoon of peanut butter, or one half of a medium banana, can fit the bill perfectly. It is important to re-energize and refuel your body in order to maintain proper function and mental focus.

• Listen to what your body is telling you. When it comes to emotional snacking and eating in general, talking to yourself is actually *not* crazy. You should always ask yourself whether or not you're truly hungry, and reflect upon the reasons behind your desire to eat. Once you realize why you crave food, you can work on developing coping mechanisms that do not involve eating. (The "cookie jar" reward system that we introduced on page 28 will help you to do this.)

Remember, snacking can be a pleasurable and guilt-free experience when you plan your snacks properly. Buy the right foods, always have fruits and vegetables on hand, and don't forget to pack a healthy snack before heading out the door for work, school, or a day of golf or shopping. Eating the right snacks will make you feel more energized every day.

## WEEKLY PERSONAL GOAL

_____

_____

_____

_____

_____

_____

## WEEKLY CONCLUSION

_____

_____

_____

_____

_____

_____

_____

## MONDAY

| | FOOD | CAL. | | | | H₂O |
|---|---|---|---|---|---|---|
| **BREAKFAST** | | | | | | 🥤 |
| | | | | | | 🥤 |
| | | | | | | 🥤 |
| | | | | | | |

NOTES: _____

| | FOOD | CAL. | | | | H₂O |
|---|---|---|---|---|---|---|
| **SNACK** | | | | | | 🥤 |
| | | | | | | 🥤 |

NOTES: _____

| | FOOD | CAL. | | | | H₂O |
|---|---|---|---|---|---|---|
| **LUNCH** | | | | | | 🥤 |
| | | | | | | 🥤 |
| | | | | | | 🥤 |
| | | | | | | |

NOTES: _____

| | FOOD | CAL. | | | | H₂O |
|---|---|---|---|---|---|---|
| **SNACK** | | | | | | 🥤 |
| | | | | | | 🥤 |

NOTES: _____

| | FOOD | CAL. | | | | H₂O |
|---|---|---|---|---|---|---|
| **DINNER** | | | | | | 🥤 |
| | | | | | | 🥤 |
| | | | | | | 🥤 |
| | | | | | | |

NOTES: _____

| **SNACK** | | | | | | 🥤 |
|---|---|---|---|---|---|---|

NOTES: _____

| EXERCISE TYPE | | 15 MIN. | 30 MIN. | 45 MIN. | 60 MIN. |
|---|---|---|---|---|---|
| | | | | | |

# TUESDAY

| | FOOD | CAL. | | | | H₂O |
|---|---|---|---|---|---|---|
| **BREAKFAST** | | | | | | 🍵 |
| | | | | | | 🍵 |
| | | | | | | 🍵 |
| | | | | | | |

NOTES: _____

| | | | | | H₂O |
|---|---|---|---|---|---|
| **SNACK** | | | | | 🍵 |
| | | | | | 🍵 |

NOTES: _____

| | | | | | H₂O |
|---|---|---|---|---|---|
| **LUNCH** | | | | | 🍵 |
| | | | | | 🍵 |
| | | | | | 🍵 |
| | | | | | |

NOTES: _____

| | | | | | H₂O |
|---|---|---|---|---|---|
| **SNACK** | | | | | 🍵 |
| | | | | | 🍵 |

NOTES: _____

| | | | | | H₂O |
|---|---|---|---|---|---|
| **DINNER** | | | | | 🍵 |
| | | | | | 🍵 |
| | | | | | 🍵 |
| | | | | | |

NOTES: _____

| | | | | | |
|---|---|---|---|---|---|
| **SNACK** | | | | | 🍵 |

NOTES: 

| EXERCISE TYPE | 15 MIN. | 30 MIN. | 45 MIN. | 60 MIN. |
|---|---|---|---|---|
| | | | | |

| WEDNESDAY | FOOD | CAL. | | | | H₂O |
|---|---|---|---|---|---|---|
| **BREAKFAST** | | | | | | 🥤 |
| | | | | | | 🥤 |
| | | | | | | 🥤 |
| | | | | | | 🥤 |

NOTES: _____

| **SNACK** | | | | | | 🥤 |
|---|---|---|---|---|---|---|
| | | | | | | 🥤 |

NOTES: _____

| **LUNCH** | | | | | | 🥤 |
|---|---|---|---|---|---|---|
| | | | | | | 🥤 |
| | | | | | | 🥤 |
| | | | | | | 🥤 |

NOTES: _____

| **SNACK** | | | | | | 🥤 |
|---|---|---|---|---|---|---|
| | | | | | | 🥤 |

NOTES: _____

| **DINNER** | | | | | | 🥤 |
|---|---|---|---|---|---|---|
| | | | | | | 🥤 |
| | | | | | | 🥤 |
| | | | | | | 🥤 |

NOTES: _____

| **SNACK** | | | | | | 🥤 |
|---|---|---|---|---|---|---|

NOTES: _____

| EXERCISE TYPE | | 15 MIN. | 30 MIN. | 45 MIN. | 60 MIN. |
|---|---|---|---|---|---|
| | | | | | |

| THURSDAY | FOOD | CAL. | | | | H$_2$O |
|---|---|---|---|---|---|---|
| **BREAKFAST** | | | | | | 🥛 |
| | | | | | | 🥛 |
| | | | | | | 🥛 |
| | | | | | | |

NOTES: _____

| **SNACK** | | | | | | 🥛 |
|---|---|---|---|---|---|---|
| | | | | | | 🥛 |

NOTES: _____

| **LUNCH** | | | | | | 🥛 |
|---|---|---|---|---|---|---|
| | | | | | | 🥛 |
| | | | | | | 🥛 |
| | | | | | | |

NOTES: _____

| **SNACK** | | | | | | 🥛 |
|---|---|---|---|---|---|---|
| | | | | | | 🥛 |

NOTES: _____

| **DINNER** | | | | | | 🥛 |
|---|---|---|---|---|---|---|
| | | | | | | 🥛 |
| | | | | | | 🥛 |
| | | | | | | |

NOTES: _____

| **SNACK** | | | | | 🥛 |
|---|---|---|---|---|---|

NOTES: _____

| EXERCISE TYPE | 15 MIN. | 30 MIN. | 45 MIN. | 60 MIN. |
|---|---|---|---|---|
| | | | | |

# FRIDAY

| | FOOD | CAL. | | | | H₂O |
|---|---|---|---|---|---|---|
| **BREAKFAST** | | | | | | 🥤 |
| | | | | | | 🥤 |
| | | | | | | 🥤 |
| | | | | | | |

NOTES: _____

| | FOOD | CAL. | | | | H₂O |
|---|---|---|---|---|---|---|
| **SNACK** | | | | | | 🥤 |
| | | | | | | 🥤 |

NOTES: _____

| | FOOD | CAL. | | | | H₂O |
|---|---|---|---|---|---|---|
| **LUNCH** | | | | | | 🥤 |
| | | | | | | 🥤 |
| | | | | | | 🥤 |
| | | | | | | |

NOTES: _____

| | FOOD | CAL. | | | | H₂O |
|---|---|---|---|---|---|---|
| **SNACK** | | | | | | 🥤 |
| | | | | | | 🥤 |

NOTES: _____

| | FOOD | CAL. | | | | H₂O |
|---|---|---|---|---|---|---|
| **DINNER** | | | | | | 🥤 |
| | | | | | | 🥤 |
| | | | | | | 🥤 |
| | | | | | | |

NOTES: _____

| **SNACK** | | | | | | 🥤 |
|---|---|---|---|---|---|---|

NOTES: _____

| EXERCISE TYPE | 15 MIN. | 30 MIN. | 45 MIN. | 60 MIN. |
|---|---|---|---|---|
| | | | | |

# SATURDAY

| | FOOD | CAL. | | | | H$_2$O |
|---|---|---|---|---|---|---|
| **BREAKFAST** | | | | | | |
| | | | | | | |
| | | | | | | |
| | | | | | | |

NOTES: _____

| | | | | | | H$_2$O |
|---|---|---|---|---|---|---|
| **SNACK** | | | | | | |
| | | | | | | |

NOTES: _____

| | | | | | | H$_2$O |
|---|---|---|---|---|---|---|
| **LUNCH** | | | | | | |
| | | | | | | |
| | | | | | | |
| | | | | | | |

NOTES: _____

| | | | | | | H$_2$O |
|---|---|---|---|---|---|---|
| **SNACK** | | | | | | |
| | | | | | | |

NOTES: _____

| | | | | | | H$_2$O |
|---|---|---|---|---|---|---|
| **DINNER** | | | | | | |
| | | | | | | |
| | | | | | | |
| | | | | | | |

NOTES: _____

| | | | | | | |
|---|---|---|---|---|---|---|
| **SNACK** | | | | | | |

NOTES: _____

| EXERCISE TYPE | 15 MIN. | 30 MIN. | 45 MIN. | 60 MIN. |
|---|---|---|---|---|
| | | | | |

## SUNDAY

| | FOOD | CAL. | | | | H₂O |
|---|---|---|---|---|---|---|
| **BREAKFAST** | | | | | | 🥛 |
| | | | | | | 🥛 |
| | | | | | | 🥛 |
| | | | | | | |

NOTES:

| | | | | | | H₂O |
|---|---|---|---|---|---|---|
| **SNACK** | | | | | | 🥛 |
| | | | | | | 🥛 |

NOTES:

| | | | | | | H₂O |
|---|---|---|---|---|---|---|
| **LUNCH** | | | | | | 🥛 |
| | | | | | | 🥛 |
| | | | | | | 🥛 |
| | | | | | | |

NOTES:

| | | | | | | H₂O |
|---|---|---|---|---|---|---|
| **SNACK** | | | | | | 🥛 |
| | | | | | | 🥛 |

NOTES:

| | | | | | | H₂O |
|---|---|---|---|---|---|---|
| **DINNER** | | | | | | 🥛 |
| | | | | | | 🥛 |
| | | | | | | 🥛 |
| | | | | | | |

NOTES:

| **SNACK** | | | | | | 🥛 |
|---|---|---|---|---|---|---|

NOTES:

| EXERCISE TYPE | 15 MIN. | 30 MIN. | 45 MIN. | 60 MIN. |
|---|---|---|---|---|
| | | | | |

# Healthy Snack Options

Never again will you need to ask, "What can I eat as a snack?" We have developed a list of our favorite healthy snack options and categorized them to correspond to whatever cravings you may have. Keep in mind that this is a sampling and not a definitive list. Depending on where you live and shop, you may come across many more healthy snacks and acceptable food brands. As a general rule, snacks should be less than 200 calories, contain at least 3 grams of fiber, and provide a combination of complex carbohydrates, protein, and heart-healthy fat.

## HEALTHY SNACKS

**For when you crave something . . . CRUNCHY:** These snacks will keep you busy munching away, but remember that they must be eaten mindfully!

| SUGGESTED SNACK | OUR FAVORITE |
| --- | --- |
| **Popcorn** (100 calories each) | • 3 cups, air popped <br> • 1 Orville Redenbacher, Newman's Own, or Smart Balance 100-calorie bag |
| **Baby carrots with hummus** (115 calories total) | • 14 baby carrots (35 calories) <br> • 2 tablespoons of hummus (80 calories) |
| **Low-calorie chips** (140 calories each or less) | • 1 bag Glenny's Soy Crisps (140 calories) <br> • 1 bag Crispy Delites Natural Veggie Chips (105 calories) <br> • 14 Bachman's Multigrain Tortilla Chips (140 calories) |
| **Nuts** (170 calories each or less) | • 14 almonds or one (1) 100-calorie pack of almonds (Blue Diamond, Trader Joe's, or BJ's Wholesale) |

| **Nuts** *(cont'd.)* | • 2 tablespoons of walnuts (100 calories)<br>• 1 ounce of unsalted, natural almonds, peanuts, cashews, or pistachio nuts (See Nut Portion Guide on page 129.) |
|---|---|
| **Veggies with dip**<br>(150 calories total or less) | • 1 cup of sliced raw vegetables *or* 2 high-fiber crackers (20–50 calories)<br>• 2 tablespoons *or* 100-calorie packaged portions of guacamole or dip |
| **Snack bars**<br>(180 calories each or less) | • Kind bars, assorted varieties (180 calories or less)<br>• Gnu, assorted varieties (130 calories)<br>• Luna, assorted varieties (180 calories) |

**For when you crave something . . . SAVORY & LIGHT:**
These snacks are light, energizing, and contain just enough protein and fiber to get you through mid-afternoon slumps.

| **SUGGESTED SNACK** | **OUR FAVORITE** |
|---|---|
| **Cheese melt**<br>(135 calories total) | • ½ of a high-fiber English muffin (50 calories)<br>• 1 slice of 2% American cheese (80 calories)<br>• Sliced tomato (5 calories) |
| **Mini-pizza**<br>(175 calories total) | • Whole wheat pita (4 inches in diameter, 75 calories)<br>• 2 tablespoons of tomato sauce (30 calories)<br>• 3 tablespoons of low-fat mozzarella cheese (70 calories) |
| **Cup of soup**<br>(140 calories each or less) | • Amy's Kitchen organic low-fat black bean vegetable soup (130 calories)<br>• Healthy Choice country vegetable soup (140 calories) |

| **Hard-boiled egg and fruit** (110 calories total) | • 1 large egg (70 calories)<br>• ½ cup of berries (40 calories) |
| --- | --- |
| **Cantaloupe and cottage cheese** (140 calories total) | • ½ cup of cubed cantaloupe (40 calories)<br>• ½ cup of 2% cottage cheese (100 calories)<br>• Sprinkle with cinnamon if desired |

**For when you crave something . . . SWEET & SATISFYING:**
These snacks pack enough punch to satisfy your sweet tooth, and some have an additional bonus—disease-fighting antioxidants.

| SUGGESTED SNACK | OUR FAVORITE |
| --- | --- |
| **Frozen dessert bars and cups** (120 calories each or less) | • Edy's All Natural frozen pops, acai berry, pomegranate, strawberry, or raspberry (60-80 calories)<br>• Skinny Cow fudge pops (100 calories)<br>• ½ cup of low-fat frozen yogurt (120 calories) |
| **Low-calorie muffins** (100 calories each) | • VitaMuffins or VitaTops (Vitalicious brand) |
| **Fruit and nuts** (130 calories total) | • 1 small apple (60 calories)<br>• 10 almonds (70 calories) |
| **Low-fat cookies** (140 calories each or less) | • 30 Annie's Bunny cookies (140 calories)<br>• 15 Trader Joe's Chocolate Cat cookies (120 calories) |
| **Yogurt and berries** (150 calories total) | • 6 ounces of 0% FAGE Greek yogurt, plain (90 calories)<br>• ½ cup of blueberries (40 calories)<br>• 1 teaspoon of honey (20 calories) |
| **Dark almonds (chocolate-covered)** (100 calories total) | • Trader Joe's 80% dark chocolate almonds (6 almonds = 100 calories) |

# Goal 7

## Brighten Your Plate, Be a Healthy Weight

Let's begin with an important fact: There is no such thing as a "bad" fruit or vegetable. While some are higher in calories than others (e.g., avocados, potatoes), fruits and vegetables are full of nutrients, and most are essentially fat-free. Have you ever heard anyone claim that they gained weight by eating too many bananas?

Though undeserved, many fruits and vegetables have received a bad rap. Some fad diets have excluded fruits such as bananas and watermelon, and vegetables such as avocados, beets, carrots, and corn, for the reason that they supposedly contain too many carbohydrates and/or calories. These claims couldn't be farther from the truth. Vegetables, which average 25 calories per serving, are loaded with fiber and vitamins A and C. Many vegetables are also high in potassium (spinach, squash, celery) and calcium (spinach, broccoli, collard greens, and sweet potatoes). Likewise, fruits, which can range from 30 to 100 calories per serving, contain significant amounts of vitamins; a single serving can provide you with 100 percent of your recommended daily intake of vitamins, particularly vitamin A and vitamin C. Several fruits, especially berries, are rich in antioxidants as well, which both prevent and fight disease. One thing that fruits and vegetables are *not* loaded with is calories! Unfortunately, most people do not satisfy their daily requirements for the two most important groups on the food pyramid.

Keep a simple rule in mind as you begin to include fruits and veggies in your diet: The brighter your plate, the healthier your weight. In other words, color is a good way to gauge nutrition when it comes to fruits and vegetables. The more colorful the foods on your plate are, the more health benefits you will reap by eating them. For example, dark red vegetables contain significant amounts of beta carotene, a well-known anticarcinogenic (or cancer-fighting) nutrient. Deep green vegetables are also loaded with anticarcinogenic nutrients, and the list goes on. Still, adding *any* vegetable or fruit to your meals and snacks is an ideal way to balance your nutrition, and if you want to lose weight, manage disease, and become a healthier person overall, these foods must be incorporated into your daily eating habits.

Here is some practical advice for increasing your intake of fruits and vegetables. Follow these tips, and they will become a basic and indispensable part of your lifestyle.

☑ **Include fruits and vegetables with every meal.** Start your day with a piece of fruit to accompany your toast or eggs, or sprinkle berries on top of your cereal. At lunch, eat a salad or pack baby carrots, celery sticks, or a serving of vegetable or bean soup to eat with your sandwich. Start dinner with one half of a grapefruit or melon, and end the meal with a salad. Vegetables should also be a dinner staple, whether steamed, roasted, grilled, sautéed, or raw.

☑ **Eat fruits and vegetables as snacks.** A piece of fruit makes a great snack, especially if you're always on the go. Other options include a yogurt parfait with berries; apple slices spread with a tablespoon of peanut butter; or chopped veggies with hummus or another low-fat dip. See our snack chart in Goal 6 on pages 98 to 100.

☑️ **Build a salad.** A well-built salad can meet your vegetable requirements for the day depending on the size and the veggies it includes. Make it interesting: Include as many vegetables as you can to add volume and color. You may even choose to add fruits such as berries, cubed apple, grapefruit sections, and sliced pear or mango, all of which go nicely in the right salad. Our guide, which begins on page 112, will give you more salad ideas.

☑️ **Eat a rainbow.** If you buy more colorful fruits and vegetables, you'll avoid falling into a rut and becoming bored with your meals. Eating a wide variety of colors will allow you to consume a wide variety of nutrients and keep it interesting all at once.

☑️ **Become an omelet enthusiast.** Omelets are already a great source of protein, but you can make them a great source of vegetables too. Adding peppers, spinach, artichokes, and mushrooms to your eggs will both spruce up your meal and give you a perfect combination of protein and veggies. You can also fit in a serving of fruit by chopping up a tomato in your omelet.

☑️ **Keep fruits and veggies on hand.** Try to buy fresh produce more than once a week, and buy only a few days' worth to prevent waste. Also, keeping a supply of frozen fruits and vegetables in your freezer will come in handy when you want to make a quick stir-fry, vegetable omelet, side dish, or smoothie. Fruits and vegetables are frozen at the peak of their ripeness and are usually optimal in their nutrient density. When it comes to dried fruit, however, it's best to eat it sparingly since it is calorically dense.

☑️ **Strive for 5 to 9.** Consume a total of *5 to 9* fruits and vegetables each day (try to go heavier with vegetables than fruit), and watch your weight melt away. You may remember from Goal 2 that a serving of fruit or vegetables varies from

½ to 1 cup, which can also be measured as an open handful or a fist. Refer to your log and pay attention to the number of fruits and vegetables you are consuming. When you focus on fitting in the recommended amount of veggie and fruit servings, you may be forced to eliminate other higher-calorie foods from your diet. Drinking enough water will reduce unpleasant side effects of eating vegetables in bulk, such as excess gas and bloating.

The benefits of increasing the amount of fruits and vegetables you eat extend far beyond weight loss. They also make you feel and look healthier, boost your energy and immunity, prevent chronic disease, and improve your overall health.

**WEEKLY PERSONAL GOAL**

**WEEKLY CONCLUSION**

## MONDAY

| | FOOD | CAL. | | | | H$_2$O |
|---|---|---|---|---|---|---|
| **BREAKFAST** | | | | | | 🍵 |
| | | | | | | 🍵 |
| | | | | | | 🍵 |
| | | | | | | |

NOTES:

| | FOOD | CAL. | | | | H$_2$O |
|---|---|---|---|---|---|---|
| **SNACK** | | | | | | 🍵 |
| | | | | | | 🍵 |

NOTES:

| | FOOD | CAL. | | | | H$_2$O |
|---|---|---|---|---|---|---|
| **LUNCH** | | | | | | 🍵 |
| | | | | | | 🍵 |
| | | | | | | 🍵 |

NOTES:

| | FOOD | CAL. | | | | H$_2$O |
|---|---|---|---|---|---|---|
| **SNACK** | | | | | | 🍵 |
| | | | | | | 🍵 |

NOTES:

| | FOOD | CAL. | | | | H$_2$O |
|---|---|---|---|---|---|---|
| **DINNER** | | | | | | 🍵 |
| | | | | | | 🍵 |
| | | | | | | 🍵 |

NOTES:

| | | | | | | |
|---|---|---|---|---|---|---|
| **SNACK** | | | | | | 🍵 |

NOTES:

| EXERCISE TYPE | 15 MIN. | 30 MIN. | 45 MIN. | 60 MIN. |
|---|---|---|---|---|
| | | | | |

# TUESDAY

| | FOOD | CAL. | | | | H₂O |
|---|---|---|---|---|---|---|
| **BREAKFAST** | | | | | | 🥤 |
| | | | | | | 🥤 |
| | | | | | | 🥤 |
| | | | | | | |

NOTES: _____

| | | | | | | H₂O |
|---|---|---|---|---|---|---|
| **SNACK** | | | | | | 🥤 |
| | | | | | | 🥤 |

NOTES: _____

| | | | | | | H₂O |
|---|---|---|---|---|---|---|
| **LUNCH** | | | | | | 🥤 |
| | | | | | | 🥤 |
| | | | | | | 🥤 |

NOTES: _____

| | | | | | | H₂O |
|---|---|---|---|---|---|---|
| **SNACK** | | | | | | 🥤 |
| | | | | | | 🥤 |

NOTES: _____

| | | | | | | H₂O |
|---|---|---|---|---|---|---|
| **DINNER** | | | | | | 🥤 |
| | | | | | | 🥤 |
| | | | | | | 🥤 |

NOTES: _____

| | | | | | | |
|---|---|---|---|---|---|---|
| **SNACK** | | | | | | 🥤 |

NOTES: _____

| EXERCISE TYPE | 15 MIN. | 30 MIN. | 45 MIN. | 60 MIN. |
|---|---|---|---|---|
| | | | | |

| WEDNESDAY | FOOD | CAL. | | | | H₂O |
|---|---|---|---|---|---|---|
| **BREAKFAST** | | | | | | 🥤 |
| | | | | | | 🥤 |
| | | | | | | 🥤 |
| | | | | | | |

NOTES: _____

| **SNACK** | | | | | | 🥤 |
|---|---|---|---|---|---|---|
| | | | | | | 🥤 |

NOTES: _____

| **LUNCH** | | | | | | 🥤 |
|---|---|---|---|---|---|---|
| | | | | | | 🥤 |
| | | | | | | 🥤 |
| | | | | | | |

NOTES: _____

| **SNACK** | | | | | | 🥤 |
|---|---|---|---|---|---|---|
| | | | | | | 🥤 |

NOTES: _____

| **DINNER** | | | | | | 🥤 |
|---|---|---|---|---|---|---|
| | | | | | | 🥤 |
| | | | | | | 🥤 |
| | | | | | | |

NOTES: _____

| **SNACK** | | | | | | 🥤 |
|---|---|---|---|---|---|---|

NOTES: _____

| EXERCISE TYPE | 15 MIN. | 30 MIN. | 45 MIN. | 60 MIN. |
|---|---|---|---|---|
| | | | | |

## THURSDAY

| | FOOD | CAL. | | | | H₂O |
|---|---|---|---|---|---|---|
| **BREAKFAST** | | | | | | 🥤 |
| | | | | | | 🥤 |
| | | | | | | 🥤 |
| | | | | | | |

NOTES: _____

| | FOOD | CAL. | | | | H₂O |
|---|---|---|---|---|---|---|
| **SNACK** | | | | | | 🥤 |
| | | | | | | 🥤 |

NOTES: _____

| | FOOD | CAL. | | | | H₂O |
|---|---|---|---|---|---|---|
| **LUNCH** | | | | | | 🥤 |
| | | | | | | 🥤 |
| | | | | | | 🥤 |
| | | | | | | |

NOTES: _____

| | FOOD | CAL. | | | | H₂O |
|---|---|---|---|---|---|---|
| **SNACK** | | | | | | 🥤 |
| | | | | | | 🥤 |

NOTES: _____

| | FOOD | CAL. | | | | H₂O |
|---|---|---|---|---|---|---|
| **DINNER** | | | | | | 🥤 |
| | | | | | | 🥤 |
| | | | | | | 🥤 |
| | | | | | | |

NOTES: _____

| **SNACK** | | | | | 🥤 |
|---|---|---|---|---|---|

NOTES: _____

| EXERCISE TYPE | 15 MIN. | 30 MIN. | 45 MIN. | 60 MIN. |
|---|---|---|---|---|
| | | | | |

| FRIDAY | FOOD | CAL. | | | | H₂O |
|---|---|---|---|---|---|---|
| **BREAKFAST** | | | | | | 🥛 |
| | | | | | | |
| | | | | | | 🥛 |
| | | | | | | 🥛 |

NOTES:

| **SNACK** | | | | | | 🥛 |
|---|---|---|---|---|---|---|
| | | | | | | 🥛 |

NOTES:

| **LUNCH** | | | | | | 🥛 |
|---|---|---|---|---|---|---|
| | | | | | | |
| | | | | | | 🥛 |
| | | | | | | 🥛 |

NOTES:

| **SNACK** | | | | | | 🥛 |
|---|---|---|---|---|---|---|
| | | | | | | 🥛 |

NOTES:

| **DINNER** | | | | | | 🥛 |
|---|---|---|---|---|---|---|
| | | | | | | |
| | | | | | | 🥛 |
| | | | | | | 🥛 |

NOTES:

| **SNACK** | | | | | | 🥛 |
|---|---|---|---|---|---|---|

NOTES:

| EXERCISE TYPE | | 15 MIN. | 30 MIN. | 45 MIN. | 60 MIN. |
|---|---|---|---|---|---|
| | | | | | |

## SATURDAY

| | FOOD | CAL. | | | | H₂O |
|---|---|---|---|---|---|---|
| **BREAKFAST** | | | | | | 🥤 🥤 🥤 |

NOTES: _____

| | | | | | | H₂O |
|---|---|---|---|---|---|---|
| **SNACK** | | | | | | 🥤 🥤 |

NOTES: _____

| | | | | | | H₂O |
|---|---|---|---|---|---|---|
| **LUNCH** | | | | | | 🥤 🥤 🥤 |

NOTES: _____

| | | | | | | H₂O |
|---|---|---|---|---|---|---|
| **SNACK** | | | | | | 🥤 🥤 |

NOTES: _____

| | | | | | | H₂O |
|---|---|---|---|---|---|---|
| **DINNER** | | | | | | 🥤 🥤 🥤 |

NOTES: _____

| | | | | | | |
|---|---|---|---|---|---|---|
| **SNACK** | | | | | | 🥤 |

NOTES: _____

| EXERCISE TYPE | 15 MIN. | 30 MIN. | 45 MIN. | 60 MIN. |
|---|---|---|---|---|
| | | | | |

## SUNDAY

| | FOOD | CAL. | | | | H$_2$O |
|---|---|---|---|---|---|---|
| **BREAKFAST** | | | | | | 🥛 |
| | | | | | | 🥛 |
| | | | | | | 🥛 |

NOTES:

| | | | | | | H$_2$O |
|---|---|---|---|---|---|---|
| **SNACK** | | | | | | 🥛 |
| | | | | | | 🥛 |

NOTES:

| | | | | | | H$_2$O |
|---|---|---|---|---|---|---|
| **LUNCH** | | | | | | 🥛 |
| | | | | | | 🥛 |
| | | | | | | 🥛 |

NOTES:

| | | | | | | H$_2$O |
|---|---|---|---|---|---|---|
| **SNACK** | | | | | | 🥛 |
| | | | | | | 🥛 |

NOTES:

| | | | | | | H$_2$O |
|---|---|---|---|---|---|---|
| **DINNER** | | | | | | 🥛 |
| | | | | | | 🥛 |
| | | | | | | 🥛 |

NOTES:

| **SNACK** | | | | | 🥛 |
|---|---|---|---|---|---|
| | | | | | |

NOTES:

| EXERCISE TYPE | | 15 MIN. | 30 MIN. | 45 MIN. | 60 MIN. |
|---|---|---|---|---|---|
| | | | | | |

# Build a Salad

A salad is one of the best ways to significantly increase your intake of vegetables—and fruits, too. Use this guide to make a salad that will meet your nutritional needs and satisfy your appetite without expanding your waist size. We have also included calorie amounts for salad ingredients and dressings that are higher in calories and fat. This way, you will have the information necessary to make a nutritious salad that will not sabotage your efforts to be healthy. Some ingredients are too often used as salad *staples* rather than salad *extras*. Although it is unnecessary to completely eliminate them from your diet, use these extras in small amounts and only as an occasional treat.

## A Guide to Building Your Salad

**1.** Start with 3 cups of lettuce. The darker the green the better.

| LETTUCE | CALORIES (PER CUP) |
| --- | --- |
| Arugula | 5 |
| Baby spinach | 7 |
| Mesculin/mixed greens | 15 |
| Romaine | 10 |
| Watercress | 4 |

**2.** Add vegetables. You are not restricted to the ones listed here.

| VEGETABLE | CALORIES (PER ¼ CUP) |
| --- | --- |
| Artichoke hearts | 9 |
| Asparagus | 10 |
| Beets | 15 |
| Bell pepper | 7 |
| Broccoli | 14 |

| VEGETABLE *(continued)* | CALORIES (PER ¼ CUP) |
|---|---|
| Carrots | 11 |
| Celery | 4 |
| Cucumbers | 5 |
| Hearts of palm | 12 |
| Mushrooms | 4 |
| Red onions | 12 |
| Tomatoes | 8 |

**3.** Add higher-calorie vegetable and legumes. Limit your total to ¼ cup.

| VEGETABLE/LEGUME | CALORIES (PER ¼ CUP) |
|---|---|
| Chickpeas (Garbanzo beans) | 71 |
| Corn | 33 |
| Edamame | 64 |
| Peas | 34 |
| Red kidney beans | 54 |

**4.** Add a protein. Four to six ounces are recommended.

| PROTEIN | CALORIES (PER 2 OZ.) |
|---|---|
| Chicken, grilled | 60 |
| Egg, 1 whole | 75 |
| Egg white, 1 | 17 |
| Tofu | 91 |
| Tuna, in water and drained | 50 |
| Turkey, roasted | 50 |
| Salmon, canned | 80 |
| Salmon, grilled | 122 |

| PROTEIN *(continued)* | CALORIES (PER 2 OZ.) |
|---|---|
| Sardines, in oil and drained | 120 |
| Shrimp, grilled | 60 |
| Veggie burger, frozen | 100-120 |

**5.** Add a serving of fat. Use cheese sparingly and occasionally.

| FAT | CALORIES |
|---|---|
| Almonds (½ oz. or 14 nuts) | 85 |
| Avocado (1 oz. or 3 slices) | 50 |
| Cheese, bleu cheese (1 oz.) | 100 |
| Cheese, cheddar (1 oz.) | 114 |
| Cheese, feta (1 oz.) | 75 |
| Cheese, goat (1 oz.) | 106 |
| Cheese, mozzarella (1 oz.) | 86 |
| Cheese, parmesan (1 oz.) | 110 |
| Olives | |
|    Black (8 large) | 45 |
|    Green (10 large) | 45 |
| Olive oil (1 tsp) | 40 |
| Walnuts (½ oz. or 8 halves) | 93 |

**6.** If you wish, add fruit or other extras—but cautiously. We have included extras like bacon and croutons to make you aware of how many calories you may potentially add to your otherwise low-calorie salad.

| EXTRA | CALORIES (PER ¼ CUP) |
|---|---|
| Apple | 14 |
| Bacon (2 oz.) | 160 |

| EXTRA *(continued)* | CALORIES (PER ¼ CUP) |
|---|---|
| Craisins | 117 |
| Croutons (2 scoops) | 120 |
| Orange slices | 20 |
| Oriental noodles (2 tbsp.) | 35 |
| Raisins | 108 |

**7.** Add a limited amount of dressing—no more than 1 to 2 tablespoons for most dressings, and slightly more if you are using vinegar. Opt for oil-based dressings or vinaigrette over creamy dressings. Also, it is preferable to use olive oil or low-fat dressings over fat-free, as fat helps absorb nutrients in the salad.

| DRESSING | CALORIES (PER 1 TBSP.) |
|---|---|
| Balsamic vinaigrette | 55 |
| Balsamic vinegar | 10 |
| Bleu cheese | 77 |
| Caesar | 78 |
| Honey mustard | 60 |
| Oil and vinegar | 55 |
| Ranch | 75 |

**FREEBIES TO ADD:**

| | | |
|---|---|---|
| • Herbs | • Mustard | • Spices |
| • Lemon | • Salsa | • Vinegar |

Eat it whole or chop it. Serve it on a plate or in a big glass bowl. Have it with your meal or as your meal. Be creative and, most importantly, enjoy it!

# Goal 8

## Fat—Eat It Without Being It

**I**f you're like most people, you know that consuming a large quantity of foods high in fat will probably cause you to gain weight. However, the right fats are an essential part of a well-balanced diet. So what do you do?

For starters, you should understand that there are desirable fats and undesirable fats. Desirable fats include monounsaturated fats (olive oil, nuts/seeds, avocados, dark chocolate) and polyunsaturated fats (vegetable oils such as safflower, corn, sunflower, soy, and canola). An omega-3 is an exceptionally healthy type of polyunsaturated fat found in salmon, walnuts, flaxseed, and flaxseed oil. These "good" fats should be consumed daily, but only in small quantities; in this case, there *can* be too much of a good thing.

The less desirable fats should *not* be consumed on a daily basis, and some should even be avoided altogether. Saturated fats, which are found in animal products such as butter, whole milk, steak, and ice cream can be eaten in small amounts, but you should refrain from eating any food that contains trans fat. When consumed regularly, trans fat—manufactured fat found mainly in packaged and processed foods—leads to weight gain and can put you at risk for diabetes, high cholesterol, and heart disease. Most

nutrition labels indicate if trans fat is present in the food—
look for the terms "hydrogenated" or "partially hydrogenated" on the list of ingredients.

As long as you limit your portion size, healthy fats
greatly improve your nutritional well-being and help you
to manage your weight. Though high in calories, desirable
fat is a necessary part of a balanced diet and should become
a staple in your new healthy lifestyle. Your goal this week is
to include one to three servings of healthy fats (in con-
trolled portions) at each meal or snack.

Here are some ways you can incorporate desirable fats
into your diet in appropriate amounts:

• **Eat a serving of nuts or seeds daily.** Nuts make a great
healthy snack, but, as with most foods, overindulging can
work against your weight loss goals. Watch your portion
size and avoid the temptation to overeat by purchasing 100-
calorie packs and nut bars, or by measuring properly sized
servings from a larger container to store in individual plastic bags. You can also incorporate nuts into your diet by
sprinkling them in salads and stir-fry, or by spreading a
small amount of nut butter (almond, peanut, sunflower,
etc.) on a piece of fruit or high-fiber cracker. To determine
correct portion sizes for different types of nuts, refer to our
Nut Portion Guide on page 129.

• **Keep it interesting: Use oil.** Using oil to cook, prepare, or
flavor your food is a good way to spice up your meals without overloading them with empty calories. Oils can be
added to pasta, stir-fry dishes, and marinades, or used to
coat vegetables and dress salads. Whether olive, canola, avocado, sesame, or oils made from peanuts, walnuts, or
macadamias, oil should be used in moderation. One teaspoon per meal is a sufficient amount.

• **Include fatty fish in your diet.** Eating salmon is a great way to do this, especially since it contains the most omega-3's, a "good" fat with several health benefits. Omega-3 fatty acids reduce inflammation, and there is evidence that suggests they also help lower the risk of chronic diseases such as heart disease, cancer, and arthritis. Omega-3 fats are also highly concentrated in the brain and appear to improve cognitive and behavioral functions like memory. In addition to salmon, fish that contain significant amounts of omega-3 fat include halibut, herring, mackerel, and sardines. Try to eat fatty fish twice a week.

• **Dress your salad.** A light coating of dressing on your salad will not only add flavor, but also facilitate the absorption of nutrients. The healthiest way to dress your salad is to mix 1 teaspoon to 1 tablespoon of olive oil with vinegar, herbs (either fresh or dried), and fresh lemon juice. If you use a prepared dressing, 1 tablespoon of vinaigrette or 2 tablespoons of reduced fat dressing is acceptable. Avoid creamy salad dressings such as Caesar, ranch, and bleu cheese, as these usually contain unhealthy saturated fats.

• **Embrace avocados.** Avocados are a unique fruit because they contain monounsaturated fat, which provides nutritional benefits when consumed in moderation. Avocados can be added to salads, sliced and put on sandwiches (we love turkey and avocado on rye), and used in salsa toppings for chicken or fish. Two tablespoons of guacamole dip with veggies also makes a tasty and satisfying snack.

• **Don't cut out chocolate.** Yes, you read that correctly. Dark chocolate with a cocoa content of 70 percent or greater contains monounsaturated fat and makes a delicious evening snack that will satisfy your sweet tooth. Again, make sure you only eat dark chocolate in small portions, especially since it can be very tempting to overeat. For help with figuring out correct portion sizes, refer to our Portion Control Guide on page 46.

Adding desirable fat to your daily diet in small amounts can have big results. "Good" fats promote brain and heart health as well as prevent your risk of diabetes and certain cancers. Additionally, healthy fats are a crucial part of any dietary regimen, since they keep meals and snacks both balanced and satisfying. Evidence has also shown that including healthy fats in your diet decreases belly fat. So mindfully eat fat to lose fat!

## WEEKLY PERSONAL GOAL

_____

_____

_____

_____

_____

## WEEKLY CONCLUSION

_____

_____

_____

_____

_____

## MONDAY

| | FOOD | CAL. | | | | H$_2$O |
|---|---|---|---|---|---|---|
| **BREAKFAST** | | | | | | 🥤 |
| | | | | | | 🥤 |
| | | | | | | 🥤 |
| | | | | | | |

NOTES:

| | FOOD | CAL. | | | | H$_2$O |
|---|---|---|---|---|---|---|
| **SNACK** | | | | | | 🥤 |
| | | | | | | 🥤 |

NOTES:

| | FOOD | CAL. | | | | H$_2$O |
|---|---|---|---|---|---|---|
| **LUNCH** | | | | | | 🥤 |
| | | | | | | 🥤 |
| | | | | | | 🥤 |
| | | | | | | |

NOTES:

| | FOOD | CAL. | | | | H$_2$O |
|---|---|---|---|---|---|---|
| **SNACK** | | | | | | 🥤 |
| | | | | | | 🥤 |

NOTES:

| | FOOD | CAL. | | | | H$_2$O |
|---|---|---|---|---|---|---|
| **DINNER** | | | | | | 🥤 |
| | | | | | | 🥤 |
| | | | | | | 🥤 |
| | | | | | | |

NOTES:

| **SNACK** | | | | | 🥤 |
|---|---|---|---|---|---|

NOTES:

| EXERCISE TYPE | 15 MIN. | 30 MIN. | 45 MIN. | 60 MIN. |
|---|---|---|---|---|
| | | | | |

## TUESDAY

| | FOOD | CAL. | | | | H$_2$O |
|---|---|---|---|---|---|---|
| **BREAKFAST** | | | | | | 🥤 |
| | | | | | | 🥤 |
| | | | | | | 🥤 |
| | | | | | | |

NOTES: _____

| | | | | | | H$_2$O |
|---|---|---|---|---|---|---|
| **SNACK** | | | | | | 🥤 |
| | | | | | | 🥤 |

NOTES: _____

| | | | | | | |
|---|---|---|---|---|---|---|
| **LUNCH** | | | | | | 🥤 |
| | | | | | | 🥤 |
| | | | | | | 🥤 |

NOTES: _____

| | | | | | | |
|---|---|---|---|---|---|---|
| **SNACK** | | | | | | 🥤 |
| | | | | | | 🥤 |

NOTES: _____

| | | | | | | |
|---|---|---|---|---|---|---|
| **DINNER** | | | | | | 🥤 |
| | | | | | | 🥤 |
| | | | | | | 🥤 |

NOTES: _____

| | | | | | | |
|---|---|---|---|---|---|---|
| **SNACK** | | | | | | 🥤 |

NOTES: _____

| EXERCISE TYPE | 15 MIN. | 30 MIN. | 45 MIN. | 60 MIN. |
|---|---|---|---|---|
| | | | | |

## WEDNESDAY

| | FOOD | CAL. | | | | H₂O |
|---|---|---|---|---|---|---|
| **BREAKFAST** | | | | | | 🥤 🥤 🥤 |

NOTES: _____

| | FOOD | CAL. | | | | H₂O |
|---|---|---|---|---|---|---|
| **SNACK** | | | | | | 🥤 🥤 |

NOTES: _____

| | FOOD | CAL. | | | | H₂O |
|---|---|---|---|---|---|---|
| **LUNCH** | | | | | | 🥤 🥤 🥤 |

NOTES: _____

| | FOOD | CAL. | | | | H₂O |
|---|---|---|---|---|---|---|
| **SNACK** | | | | | | 🥤 🥤 |

NOTES: _____

| | FOOD | CAL. | | | | H₂O |
|---|---|---|---|---|---|---|
| **DINNER** | | | | | | 🥤 🥤 🥤 |

NOTES: _____

| **SNACK** | | | | | | 🥤 |
|---|---|---|---|---|---|---|

NOTES: _____

| EXERCISE TYPE | 15 MIN. | 30 MIN. | 45 MIN. | 60 MIN. |
|---|---|---|---|---|
| | | | | |

## THURSDAY

| | FOOD | CAL. | | | | H₂O |
|---|---|---|---|---|---|---|
| **BREAKFAST** | | | | | | ⛾ |
| | | | | | | ⛾ |
| | | | | | | ⛾ |
| | | | | | | |

NOTES: _____

| | | | | | H₂O |
|---|---|---|---|---|---|
| **SNACK** | | | | | ⛾ |
| | | | | | ⛾ |

NOTES: _____

| | | | | | H₂O |
|---|---|---|---|---|---|
| **LUNCH** | | | | | ⛾ |
| | | | | | ⛾ |
| | | | | | ⛾ |
| | | | | | |

NOTES: _____

| | | | | | H₂O |
|---|---|---|---|---|---|
| **SNACK** | | | | | ⛾ |
| | | | | | ⛾ |

NOTES: _____

| | | | | | H₂O |
|---|---|---|---|---|---|
| **DINNER** | | | | | ⛾ |
| | | | | | ⛾ |
| | | | | | ⛾ |
| | | | | | |

NOTES: _____

| | | | | | |
|---|---|---|---|---|---|
| **SNACK** | | | | | ⛾ |

NOTES: _____

| EXERCISE TYPE | 15 MIN. | 30 MIN. | 45 MIN. | 60 MIN. |
|---|---|---|---|---|
| | | | | |

| FRIDAY | FOOD | CAL. | | | | H₂O |
|---|---|---|---|---|---|---|
| **BREAKFAST** | | | | | | 🥛 |
| | | | | | | 🥛 |
| | | | | | | 🥛 |
| | | | | | | 🥛 |

NOTES: _____

| **SNACK** | | | | | | 🥛 |
|---|---|---|---|---|---|---|
| | | | | | | 🥛 |

NOTES: _____

| **LUNCH** | | | | | | 🥛 |
|---|---|---|---|---|---|---|
| | | | | | | 🥛 |
| | | | | | | 🥛 |
| | | | | | | 🥛 |

NOTES: _____

| **SNACK** | | | | | | 🥛 |
|---|---|---|---|---|---|---|
| | | | | | | 🥛 |

NOTES: _____

| **DINNER** | | | | | | 🥛 |
|---|---|---|---|---|---|---|
| | | | | | | 🥛 |
| | | | | | | 🥛 |
| | | | | | | 🥛 |

NOTES: _____

| **SNACK** | | | | | 🥛 |
|---|---|---|---|---|---|

NOTES: _____

| EXERCISE TYPE | 15 MIN. | 30 MIN. | 45 MIN. | 60 MIN. |
|---|---|---|---|---|
| | | | | |

| SATURDAY | FOOD | CAL. | | | | H₂O |
|---|---|---|---|---|---|---|
| **BREAKFAST** | | | | | | 🥤 |
| | | | | | | 🥤 |
| | | | | | | 🥤 |
| | | | | | | |

NOTES:

| **SNACK** | | | | | | 🥤 |
|---|---|---|---|---|---|---|
| | | | | | | 🥤 |

NOTES:

| **LUNCH** | | | | | | 🥤 |
|---|---|---|---|---|---|---|
| | | | | | | 🥤 |
| | | | | | | 🥤 |
| | | | | | | |

NOTES:

| **SNACK** | | | | | | 🥤 |
|---|---|---|---|---|---|---|
| | | | | | | 🥤 |

NOTES:

| **DINNER** | | | | | | 🥤 |
|---|---|---|---|---|---|---|
| | | | | | | 🥤 |
| | | | | | | 🥤 |
| | | | | | | |

NOTES:

| **SNACK** | | | | | 🥤 |
|---|---|---|---|---|---|

NOTES:

| EXERCISE TYPE | 15 MIN. | 30 MIN. | 45 MIN. | 60 MIN. |
|---|---|---|---|---|
| | | | | |

## SUNDAY

| | FOOD | CAL. | | | | H₂O |
|---|---|---|---|---|---|---|
| **BREAKFAST** | | | | | | 🥛 |
| | | | | | | 🥛 |
| | | | | | | 🥛 |
| | | | | | | |

NOTES: _____

| | | | | | | H₂O |
|---|---|---|---|---|---|---|
| **SNACK** | | | | | | 🥛 |
| | | | | | | 🥛 |

NOTES: _____

| | | | | | | H₂O |
|---|---|---|---|---|---|---|
| **LUNCH** | | | | | | 🥛 |
| | | | | | | 🥛 |
| | | | | | | 🥛 |

NOTES: _____

| | | | | | | H₂O |
|---|---|---|---|---|---|---|
| **SNACK** | | | | | | 🥛 |
| | | | | | | 🥛 |

NOTES: _____

| | | | | | | H₂O |
|---|---|---|---|---|---|---|
| **DINNER** | | | | | | 🥛 |
| | | | | | | 🥛 |
| | | | | | | 🥛 |

NOTES: _____

| | | | | | | H₂O |
|---|---|---|---|---|---|---|
| **SNACK** | | | | | | 🥛 |

NOTES: _____

| EXERCISE TYPE | 15 MIN. | 30 MIN. | 45 MIN. | 60 MIN. |
|---|---|---|---|---|
| | | | | |

# How to Eat Nuts
# Without Going Nuts!

You have probably heard the familiar saying, "Eat everything in moderation." This definitely rings true when it comes to eating nuts on a daily basis. As with any calorically dense food, overindulging in nuts—despite their nutritional value—will cause the pounds to pile on. However, when nuts are eaten mindfully, you will gain vital nutrients rather than weight. One serving of nuts a day is all it takes to curb your appetite and reduce your risk of heart disease and high blood pressure. In addition, it has been proven that people who eat a single serving of nuts each day will weigh less.

The only downside to nuts is their oil content, which will cause them to go rancid quickly if they are not stored properly. Keep them in a container in your fridge or freezer to preserve their freshness for as long as two years, and always have an ideal snack on hand. A small portion of nuts and a piece of fruit makes for a balanced combination of protein, fiber, and healthy fat that will also satisfy your sweet tooth. For example, pair one small apple with ten almonds or a pear with six walnut halves.

Due to their small size and tendency to be packaged and sold in large containers, nuts are often consumed many cups or handfuls at a time—which can add up to hundreds of calories. To gain optimal benefits from their nutrients, stick to an appropriate serving size of 1 ounce or ¼ cup (think one shot glass' worth), either at one sitting or spread out over the course of the day, and paired with other snack foods such as fruit or yogurt. The Nut Portion Guide will help you avoid overindulgence by allowing you to visualize proper portions of various types of nuts. The amount you consume each day will also depend on your hunger/fullness levels and overall calorie intake, but use this chart as a reference starting point, and begin to eat nuts to replace other fats in your diet.

## Nut Portion Guide

| NUTS | NO. OF NUTS IN 1 OUNCE | CALORIES PER OUNCE |
| --- | --- | --- |
| Almonds | 28 | 170 |
| Cashews | 18 | 160 |
| Hazelnuts | 20 | 175 |
| Macadamias | 10-12 | 205 |
| Peanuts | 28 | 165 |
| Pecans, halves | 20 | 200 |
| Pine nuts | 150-157 | 190 |
| Pistachios | 49 | 170 |
| Walnuts, halves | 14 | 185 |

We have not included Brazil nuts in the portion guide due to their high selenium content, a mineral that becomes toxic when consumed in excess. Although selenium has powerful antioxidant properties and works against aging, tissue damage, and other diseases, too much of it can produce side effects such as rashes and brittle nails. For this reason, we recommend eating no more than one or two Brazil nuts per day, which will provide you with plenty of cancer-fighting nutrients.

# Uncle Sam Wants You . . . To Eat Better

In 2011, the United States Department of Agriculture (USDA) and Health and Human Services (HHS) released the revised *Dietary Guidelines for Americans*, a set of practical nutritional recommendations for Americans ages two and older. The guidelines are updated every five years to help people make informed food choices, manage their weight, and achieve better overall health. The revised suggestions address the growing rate of obesity among children and adults, with stronger emphasis on increased physical activity and decreased calorie intake. Because the official report is several hundred pages, we have highlighted some of its most important points below:

• Avoid oversized portions.

• Choose foods that contain the least amount of sodium, and cut your overall sodium intake to less than 1,500 milligrams per day.

• Consume fewer calories during the day, particularly by decreasing your intake of foods containing solid fats and added sugars, as well as refined grains (white bread, cookies, pastries).

• Drink water instead of sugary beverages.

• Eat seafood twice a week.

• Enjoy your food, but eat less.

• Make half of your plate fruits and vegetables.

• Participate in moderate physical activity for thirty minutes most days of the week.

• Shift to a diet consisting mainly of vegetables, fruits, whole grains, nuts, beans, and seeds.

• Switch to fat-free or low-fat (1 percent) milk and milk products.

By incorporating these guidelines into your lifestyle, you will maximize the nutritional value of your meals and gain control of your weight and overall health.

# Goal 9

## Master the Menu

Restaurant menus make it difficult to stick to a nutrition plan, and most restaurants have a single objective: They want you to order an appetizer, an entrée, and a dessert, and then wash it all down with a high-calorie (and preferably high-priced) beverage. The driving force behind any restaurant is customer satisfaction, so naturally they are more concerned with taste than with health. This explains why restaurant cuisine is typically served in extra-large portions, cooked in unhealthy oils, and loaded with salt and other fattening ingredients. Restaurants are businesses, so they want you to keep coming back for more—and their goal is at odds with *your* goal.

However, it's possible to eat at a restaurant without overeating or only eating foods that are extremely high in calories—you *can* still be healthy! Here are some hints for staying on course when it comes to ordering a main course off a menu.

• **Snack at home before heading out.** If you eat a healthy snack before you go to a restaurant, you're more likely to make a sensible choice when ordering your meal. Combining an expansive, appealing menu with an empty stomach is a recipe for poor food choices, so curb your hunger by eating veggies or fruit with an ounce of protein (i.e., an apple and a hard-boiled egg) before leaving your house.

• **Know the keywords to look for.** Meal descriptions on the menu usually indicate how food is prepared, and there are certain "keywords" that will allow you to distinguish between healthy and unhealthy options. Words like *steamed*, *broiled*, *grilled*, *poached*, or *baked* generally signal healthier choices, but when in doubt, don't be afraid to ask your server how a meal is prepared. Also keep in mind that many larger chain restaurants now specify low-calorie and low-fat options on their menus, and many more post nutritional information on their websites.

• **Know the keywords to avoid.** Any meal description that contains the words *au gratin* (read: covered in breadcrumbs and cheese), *crispy*, *cheesy*, *cream sauce*, *pink sauce*, *fried*, *butter*, and *jumbo* are red flags. Avoid these unhealthy high-calorie meals. Remember that red sauce and grated parmesan cheese are healthier (but equally tasty) alternatives to pink sauce and melted or fried cheese.

• **Pay attention to the size of the portion you are served.** If you know the portion is too large for one person (and they usually are), share it with someone at your table or bring half of it home with you. Many appetizers and sides provide plenty of food and are probably closer to correct serving sizes, so consider ordering an appetizer as a main course and add a side of vegetables. You can also replace an oversized entrée with two healthy appetizers, such as a salad and a bowl of mussels.

• **Avoid the breadbasket.** Would you ever eat a huge roll before dinner at home? The answer is probably no, so don't do it when eating out either. Reaching for the breadbasket is an easy way to overload on carbohydrates and pile on calories that should be saved for your meal. You can always politely request that the basket be removed from the table, or order a starter salad so you eat veggies before your meal rather than too many carbs. Again, eating a small snack before going out to a restaurant can also help you avoid this common pitfall.

• **Use caution when it comes to ordering a salad.** Leave it to restaurants to make salads unhealthy! Whereas building your own salad at home allows you to control calorie amounts and portion sizes, ordering a salad at a restaurant is a different story, since they are notorious for packing in the calories. You should ask for your dressing and cheese on the side or for a lighter amount. In addition, avoid mayonnaise-based salad dressings (ranch, Caesar, Thousand Island, etc.) and salads loaded with "crispy" ingredients (the keywords listed above apply to salads as well). Check out our restaurant guide on pages 134 to 137 to help you make healthier choices.

• **Plan your order beforehand.** By now, you should be planning all of your meals and snacks in advance, and dining out does not have to be an exception to this habit. The internet has made restaurant menus and nutritional information accessible and available to the general public, and we encourage you to take advantage of online resources. Knowing the healthy options available to you beforehand will alleviate any stress you may have about making a smart food choice. Additionally, pre-planning your order will eliminate the temptations you might otherwise give in to, because you won't even have to open a menu at the restaurant. Refer to our guide to find delicious and nutritious options at various restaurants as well as the Calorie Guide for Chain Restaurant Foods on page 175. (Our Concession Calorie Counter on page 146 will also help you to make smarter food choices when at a sporting event or movie.) If you meet with a nutritionist, you can plan individualized meal orders for your favorite restaurants during one of your sessions.

# Staying Healthy
# While Dining Out

Picking out healthy options on a restaurant menu can be confusing and overwhelming, so we have tried to ease this burden for you. Below you will find a list of appetizers and main courses that are generally healthier and lower in calories. We have categorized our list by restaurant type so that you can make more nutritious choices at a variety of eateries. Remember to pay attention to portion size—just because it's in front of you does not mean you have to eat all of it! If you are watching your intake of sodium or carbohydrates, choose meals that are lower in salt (avoid teriyaki sauce) and starch (stay away from nachos). Also keep in mind that some larger restaurant chains offer low-calorie, low-carb, or "heart healthy" meal options on their menus. An enjoyable dinner out at a restaurant is possible—just be smart about it!

---

## BAGEL SHOP

### Breakfast

- Oatmeal
- 1 scrambled egg on a mini-bagel
- Lox and/or light cream cheese on a mini-bagel

### Lunch

- Chopped salad with no cheese, dressing on the side
- Low-fat tuna salad on a mini-bagel
- Low-fat egg white salad on a mini-bagel

---

## CHINESE

### Appetizers

- Soups: egg drop, wonton, or sweet and sour

- Any side dish of sautéed vegetables, such as string beans

**Main Courses**

- Chicken and broccoli, steamed, sauce on the side
- Chop suey
- Shrimp in black bean sauce
- Tofu and mixed vegetables
- Steamed moo shu chicken
- Steamed shrimp, chicken, or tofu with mixed vegetables, sauce on side

## DINER

- Omelet with vegetables and egg whites (add one whole egg for nutrients and satisfaction), with dry whole wheat toast or baked potato and extra veggies on the side (no hash browns)
- ¼ roasted chicken (remove skin), vegetables on the side
- Chicken souvlaki over vegetables
- Any kind of non-fried fish, vegetables on the side
- Turkey burger with lettuce and tomato, no fries
- Chopped salad of turkey, hard-boiled eggs, and vegetables over spinach or lettuce, dressing on the side (light dressing, a mix of ketchup and 1 tablespoon of mayo, or vinegar and mustard)

## ITALIAN

**Appetizers**

- Caesar salad, dressing on side (dilute the dressing with mustard and grated parmesan cheese)
- Chopped salad, dressing on side (dilute the Italian dressing with vinegar)
- Shrimp cocktail

- Mussels with marinara or white wine sauce
- Grilled portabella mushrooms or any other grilled vegetables

### Main Courses

- Shrimp marinara over spinach or any greens
- Grilled calamari, vegetables on the side
- Chicken paillard topped with grilled mushrooms
- Grilled fish, vegetables on the side
- Grilled chicken in red sauce with grated parmesan cheese (1 tablespoon), vegetables on the side
- Appetizer-sized portion of pasta with marinara sauce, or any other red sauce

---

### JAPANESE

### Appetizers

- Chicken satay
- Miso soup
- Edamame
- Salad (any kind of lettuce), dressing on side
- Naruto roll

### Main Courses

(If you are watching your sodium intake, go light on the teriyaki sauce.)

- Chicken teriyaki
- Shrimp teriyaki
- Sushi: any roll, no crunchies, not fried
  - California, salmon, or yellowtail rolls are good sushi choices
  - Order your sushi naruto style, wrapped in cucumber or brown rice

## MEXICAN

### Appetizers

- Guacamole, to be eaten with any vegetable

- Taco salad without the shell or chips,
cheese on the side. Use salsa instead of dressing.

### Main Courses

- Chicken fajitas, either in wheat tortilla
or piled over lettuce

- Shrimp fajitas, either in wheat tortilla
or piled over lettuce

- Vegetable burrito with cheese on the side, no sour cream

- Bean burrito, no sour cream or cheese

---

## STEAKHOUSE

### Appetizers

- Lettuce wedges, dressing on the side
(dilute with vinegar)

- House salad, no bacon, dressing on the side

- Shrimp cocktail

- Sautéed vegetables, light on the oil

### Main Courses

- Petite filet mignon, vegetables on the side

- Any grilled or sautéed fish, light on the oil,
vegetables on the side

- Lobster or shrimp cocktail, vegetables on the side

- Veal or lamb chops, vegetables on the side

### Sides

- Steamed or sautéed vegetables, light on the oil

- Baked potato, no sour cream or butter

The bottom line is that you have to think with your head rather than your stomach when eating at a restaurant. Prepare for a meal out by researching healthy options, planning your order, and eating a quick snack before leaving the house. In the long run, nothing will taste as good as healthiness feels. It will be well worth it to control what and how much you eat when dining out.

## WEEKLY PERSONAL GOAL

## WEEKLY CONCLUSION

# MONDAY

| | FOOD | CAL. | | | | H₂O |
|---|---|---|---|---|---|---|
| **BREAKFAST** | | | | | | 🥤 |
| | | | | | | 🥤 |
| | | | | | | 🥤 |
| | | | | | | 🥤 |

NOTES: _____

| | | | | | | H₂O |
|---|---|---|---|---|---|---|
| **SNACK** | | | | | | 🥤 |
| | | | | | | 🥤 |

NOTES: _____

| | | | | | | H₂O |
|---|---|---|---|---|---|---|
| **LUNCH** | | | | | | 🥤 |
| | | | | | | 🥤 |
| | | | | | | 🥤 |
| | | | | | | 🥤 |

NOTES: _____

| | | | | | | H₂O |
|---|---|---|---|---|---|---|
| **SNACK** | | | | | | 🥤 |
| | | | | | | 🥤 |

NOTES: _____

| | | | | | | H₂O |
|---|---|---|---|---|---|---|
| **DINNER** | | | | | | 🥤 |
| | | | | | | 🥤 |
| | | | | | | 🥤 |
| | | | | | | 🥤 |

NOTES: _____

| **SNACK** | | | | | 🥤 |
|---|---|---|---|---|---|

NOTES: _____

| EXERCISE TYPE | 15 MIN. | 30 MIN. | 45 MIN. | 60 MIN. |
|---|---|---|---|---|
| | | | | |

## TUESDAY

| | FOOD | CAL. | | | | H₂O |
|---|---|---|---|---|---|---|
| **BREAKFAST** | | | | | | 🥤 |
| | | | | | | 🥤 |
| | | | | | | 🥤 |
| | | | | | | |

NOTES: _____

| | | | | | | H₂O |
|---|---|---|---|---|---|---|
| **SNACK** | | | | | | 🥤 |
| | | | | | | 🥤 |

NOTES: _____

| | | | | | | H₂O |
|---|---|---|---|---|---|---|
| **LUNCH** | | | | | | 🥤 |
| | | | | | | 🥤 |
| | | | | | | 🥤 |

NOTES: _____

| | | | | | | H₂O |
|---|---|---|---|---|---|---|
| **SNACK** | | | | | | 🥤 |
| | | | | | | 🥤 |

NOTES: _____

| | | | | | | H₂O |
|---|---|---|---|---|---|---|
| **DINNER** | | | | | | 🥤 |
| | | | | | | 🥤 |
| | | | | | | 🥤 |

NOTES: _____

| | | | | | | H₂O |
|---|---|---|---|---|---|---|
| **SNACK** | | | | | | 🥤 |

NOTES:

| EXERCISE TYPE | 15 MIN. | 30 MIN. | 45 MIN. | 60 MIN. |
|---|---|---|---|---|
| | | | | |

| WEDNESDAY | FOOD | CAL. | | | | H₂O |
|---|---|---|---|---|---|---|
| **BREAKFAST** | | | | | | 🥛 |
| | | | | | | 🥛 |
| | | | | | | 🥛 |
| | | | | | | 🥛 |

NOTES: _____

| **SNACK** | | | | | | 🥛 |
|---|---|---|---|---|---|---|
| | | | | | | 🥛 |

NOTES: _____

| **LUNCH** | | | | | | 🥛 |
|---|---|---|---|---|---|---|
| | | | | | | 🥛 |
| | | | | | | 🥛 |
| | | | | | | 🥛 |

NOTES: _____

| **SNACK** | | | | | | 🥛 |
|---|---|---|---|---|---|---|
| | | | | | | 🥛 |

NOTES: _____

| **DINNER** | | | | | | 🥛 |
|---|---|---|---|---|---|---|
| | | | | | | 🥛 |
| | | | | | | 🥛 |
| | | | | | | 🥛 |

NOTES: _____

| **SNACK** | | | | | | 🥛 |
|---|---|---|---|---|---|---|

NOTES: _____

| EXERCISE TYPE | 15 MIN. | 30 MIN. | 45 MIN. | 60 MIN. |
|---|---|---|---|---|
| | | | | |

| THURSDAY | FOOD | CAL. | | | | $H_2O$ |
|---|---|---|---|---|---|---|
| **BREAKFAST** | | | | | | 🥤 |
| | | | | | | 🥤 |
| | | | | | | 🥤 |

NOTES: _____

| **SNACK** | | | | | | 🥤 |
|---|---|---|---|---|---|---|
| | | | | | | 🥤 |

NOTES: _____

| **LUNCH** | | | | | | 🥤 |
|---|---|---|---|---|---|---|
| | | | | | | 🥤 |
| | | | | | | 🥤 |

NOTES: _____

| **SNACK** | | | | | | 🥤 |
|---|---|---|---|---|---|---|
| | | | | | | 🥤 |

NOTES: _____

| **DINNER** | | | | | | 🥤 |
|---|---|---|---|---|---|---|
| | | | | | | 🥤 |
| | | | | | | 🥤 |

NOTES: _____

| **SNACK** | | | | | 🥤 |
|---|---|---|---|---|---|

NOTES: _____

| EXERCISE TYPE | 15 MIN. | 30 MIN. | 45 MIN. | 60 MIN. |
|---|---|---|---|---|
| | | | | |

| FRIDAY | FOOD | CAL. | | | | H$_2$O |
|---|---|---|---|---|---|---|
| **BREAKFAST** | | | | | | 🥤 |
| | | | | | | 🥤 |
| | | | | | | 🥤 |
| | | | | | | 🥤 |

NOTES: _____

| **SNACK** | | | | | | 🥤 |
|---|---|---|---|---|---|---|
| | | | | | | 🥤 |

NOTES: _____

| **LUNCH** | | | | | | 🥤 |
|---|---|---|---|---|---|---|
| | | | | | | 🥤 |
| | | | | | | 🥤 |
| | | | | | | 🥤 |

NOTES: _____

| **SNACK** | | | | | | 🥤 |
|---|---|---|---|---|---|---|
| | | | | | | 🥤 |

NOTES: _____

| **DINNER** | | | | | | 🥤 |
|---|---|---|---|---|---|---|
| | | | | | | 🥤 |
| | | | | | | 🥤 |
| | | | | | | 🥤 |

NOTES: _____

| **SNACK** | | | | | | 🥤 |
|---|---|---|---|---|---|---|

NOTES: _____

| EXERCISE TYPE | 15 MIN. | 30 MIN. | 45 MIN. | 60 MIN. |
|---|---|---|---|---|
| | | | | |

## SATURDAY

| | FOOD | CAL. | | | | H₂O |
|---|---|---|---|---|---|---|
| **BREAKFAST** | | | | | | 🥤 |
| | | | | | | 🥤 |
| | | | | | | 🥤 |
| | | | | | | |

NOTES: _____

| | | | | | | |
|---|---|---|---|---|---|---|
| **SNACK** | | | | | | 🥤 |
| | | | | | | 🥤 |

NOTES: _____

| | | | | | | |
|---|---|---|---|---|---|---|
| **LUNCH** | | | | | | 🥤 |
| | | | | | | 🥤 |
| | | | | | | 🥤 |
| | | | | | | |

NOTES: _____

| | | | | | | |
|---|---|---|---|---|---|---|
| **SNACK** | | | | | | 🥤 |
| | | | | | | 🥤 |

NOTES: _____

| | | | | | | |
|---|---|---|---|---|---|---|
| **DINNER** | | | | | | 🥤 |
| | | | | | | 🥤 |
| | | | | | | 🥤 |
| | | | | | | |

NOTES: _____

| | | | | | | |
|---|---|---|---|---|---|---|
| **SNACK** | | | | | | 🥤 |

NOTES: _____

| EXERCISE TYPE | | 15 MIN. | 30 MIN. | 45 MIN. | 60 MIN. |
|---|---|---|---|---|---|
| | | | | | |

## SUNDAY

| | FOOD | CAL. | | | | H₂O |
|---|---|---|---|---|---|---|
| **BREAKFAST** | | | | | | 🥛 |
| | | | | | | 🥛 |
| | | | | | | 🥛 |
| | | | | | | |

NOTES:

| | FOOD | CAL. | | | | H₂O |
|---|---|---|---|---|---|---|
| **SNACK** | | | | | | 🥛 |
| | | | | | | 🥛 |

NOTES:

| | FOOD | CAL. | | | | H₂O |
|---|---|---|---|---|---|---|
| **LUNCH** | | | | | | 🥛 |
| | | | | | | 🥛 |
| | | | | | | 🥛 |

NOTES:

| | FOOD | CAL. | | | | H₂O |
|---|---|---|---|---|---|---|
| **SNACK** | | | | | | 🥛 |
| | | | | | | 🥛 |

NOTES:

| | FOOD | CAL. | | | | H₂O |
|---|---|---|---|---|---|---|
| **DINNER** | | | | | | 🥛 |
| | | | | | | 🥛 |
| | | | | | | 🥛 |

NOTES:

| | FOOD | CAL. | | | | H₂O |
|---|---|---|---|---|---|---|
| **SNACK** | | | | | | 🥛 |

NOTES:

| EXERCISE TYPE | 15 MIN. | 30 MIN. | 45 MIN. | 60 MIN. |
|---|---|---|---|---|
| | | | | |

# Concession Calorie Counter

Though most concession stand complaints stem from high prices, the real problem is high calorie counts. Sporting events and movie theaters are havens for calorically dense snack foods and oversized portions. So what can you do?

First, you may want to eat a satisfying meal before you head out to the stadium or theater—enter with an empty stomach at your own risk! If your stomach isn't growling, you won't be tempted to buy a hot dog, nachos, or a bucket of buttery popcorn. Also, always practice portion control by ordering something small or splitting a snack with others. Finally, your stomach and your wallet will both benefit from sneaking in your own snack: Health bars are small enough to fit in your pocket, and those trendy oversized pocketbooks (or for men, oversized sweatshirts) might even accommodate air-popped popcorn brought from home.

The table below lists some startling calorie counts that may deter you from the concession stand next time you are at a baseball stadium or movie theater. At the very least, we hope it influences you to limit your portion size.

## Standard Stadium Snacks

| SNACK | CALORIES |
|-------|----------|
| New York pretzel | 630 |
| Zeppole | 500 |
| Cotton candy | 175 |
| Nachos, 1 large plate | 1,410 |
| Popcorn, 1 large bucket (with butter) | 2,473 |
| Chicken tenders, regular order | 810 |
| Lemonade (24 ounces) | 300 |

| | |
|---|---|
| Ice cream, soft serve (12 ounces) | 590 |
| Caramel apple | 300 |
| Nathan's grilled chicken sandwich | 380 |
| Nathan's fries (extra-large order) | 1,236 |

## Standard Movie Theater Snacks

| SNACK | CALORIES |
|---|---|
| Coke, large (24 ounces) | 290 |
| Popcorn, child-sized, no butter (5 cups) | 470 |
| Popcorn, large, no butter (20 cups) | 1,640 |
| Nachos | 715-1,100 |
| Soft pretzel | 483 |
| Junior Mints (3 ounces) | 320 |
| Starburst (24 pieces) | 480 |
| Reeses' Peanut Butter Cups (8 ounces) | 1,200 |
| Milk Duds (3 ounces) | 340 |
| Snow Caps (3 ounces) | 360 |
| Raisinets (3.5 ounces) | 380 |
| Gummy Bears (4 ounces) | 390 |
| Twizzlers (6 ounces) | 600 |

Pretty scary, right? Bringing your own snack from home will save you lots of money and even more calories, but if you do decide to buy food from the concession stand, choose wisely and drink water. If you "fall off the wagon," remember that one event isn't going to make or break your weight loss success. Just be sure to resume healthy, smart eating once the movie or baseball game has ended.

# Goal 10
## Keep on Moving

A healthy lifestyle involves keeping your body fit, and in order to improve your physical and mental well-being, you must get up and move. Your commitment to your health depends on it.

The benefits of exercise are countless. To start, exercise promotes physical wellness by boosting cardiovascular health, preventing diabetes, and strengthening your bones and muscles. Exercise also has mental and emotional benefits, as it eases stress, alleviates depression, and increases your energy. No one has ever second guessed the positive impact of physical activity on general wellness, and yet many people do not do enough of it.

The main reason for insufficient exercise is the same one often given by clients to explain why they do not eat three meals a day: Lack of time. In our fast-paced society, many people find it difficult to adjust their busy schedules in order to make time for healthy habits, and exercise is generally not high on the priority list. There is no easy or simple solution to this problem, but the goal is clear: You must make exercise a part of your daily routine. You are a priority, so exercising must be a priority as well.

Remember, every bit of physical activity counts! If three separate ten-minute walks each day are more convenient for you than one long thirty-minute walk, don't talk yourself out of it by mistakenly thinking that ten minutes is pointless. Thirty minutes of exercise spread out during the day is just as advantageous as working out for a straight thirty minutes. In fact, recent research has shown that exercise performed in segments throughout the day may be more beneficial and effective than exercising continuously one time each day.

You should also keep in mind that there are many ways to exercise, and what works for one person may not work for you. For example, while many thrive at the gym, others find it to be intimidating and more tailored to those who are already fit and toned. The only way to discover what form of exercise works for you is to try out different activities. Since research shows that you will push yourself more if you exercise with others, take an exercise class or work out with the assistance of a personal trainer. If you prefer to exercise on your own and can afford it, try using home gym equipment such as the Wii Fit, a treadmill, an elliptical machine, or a stationary bike (but don't use them for only hanging clothes). Cheaper options include small free weight sets, workout DVDs, jumping rope, or simply dancing around your house. And you aren't restricted to exercising inside—the great outdoors offers numerous options as well. Power walking, running, swimming, hiking, and tennis are all popular and fun ways to exercise, either alone or with a partner. Yoga, which can be done either indoors or outside, is an alternative form of exercise with benefits that go beyond purely physical fitness. It serves as a highly effective form of stress management and relaxation by incorporating meditation and breathing exercises.

When you move, you burn calories. So make time to exercise, find a form of exercise that you'll stick with, and keep on moving.

## CREATING A BALANCED EXERCISE PLAN

Once you decide what type of physical activity is the most enjoyable for you, you must develop a balanced exercise routine. Ideally, this will include cardiovascular exercise, weight training, and stretching so that you burn calories and fat, build muscle, and improve your flexibility. A structured plan that integrates all of these activities will allow you to achieve the balance that your body needs and, ultimately, optimal physical fitness.

Cardiovascular exercise includes running, walking, aerobics, kickboxing, swimming, bicycling, and sports such as tennis, basketball, and soccer—activities that elevate your heart rate and burn significant amounts of calories. When your goal is to lose weight, cardiovascular exercise is essential but often a daunting prospect if you do not normally exercise. If cardiovascular activity is new to you, ease your way into it by walking for thirty minutes (in total) per day. Walking is natural, simple, and safe for just about anyone. If you prefer another form of aerobic activity, start by doing ten minutes a day, three to five times a week. Gradually, you can build up to thirty minutes each day. You should always consult your physician if you're concerned about how much cardio exercise you can handle.

Weight training (or strength training) is a muscle-building form of exercise. When you increase muscle mass, you burn more fat and speed up your metabolism, which increases the rate at which you expend calories. As you age, you lose muscle mass, which slows your metabolism and makes it more difficult to lose weight. This is why weight training is so crucial: You will build and maintain muscle mass as well as prevent the loss of bone mass. Aim to do strength training exercises two to three times per week, but be careful not to overdo it at first—this will only result in injury. Start with light free weights and gradually increase the weight amount as you build your strength, and remember to take a couple days in between workouts to rest your muscles. Check out fitness websites, strength training DVDs, a gym, or the local community center to find specific exercises that will target different muscles. If this is overwhelming, the guidance and supervision of a personal trainer might be a worthwhile investment for you.

Finally, stretching regularly will enhance your flexibility by lengthening your muscles, reducing muscle tension, increasing the range of motion of joints, and boosting your circulation and energy. Stretching after exercising will also prevent injury, so remember to end your workouts with a few minutes worth of stretching. Popular and effective stretching exercises include yoga and pilates, and there are numerous classes (as well as DVDs) designed specifically for beginners that teach you modified versions of basic pilates moves and yoga poses.

Developing a balanced exercise routine will diversify the kinds of exercises you do, which counteracts boredom or lack of motivation. Don't just work to exercise—make sure exercise works for you.

## MAKE WORKING OUT WORK FOR YOU

If you don't already exercise regularly, you may find it difficult at first to make it a habit. Here are some ways you can incorporate exercise into your daily routine in ways that make it natural and fun rather than burdensome and boring.

• **Find the time.** Commit to specific days and times during which you will exercise, and stick to your schedule. As with meals, snacks, and glasses of water, planning when and how you will exercise is a key to success. If you are not regularly physically active, begin by doing ten minutes of exercise three to five times a week. As exercise becomes easier for you, work up to doing thirty minutes on each of these three to five days, and then eventually even sixty minutes, depending on your ability and level of fitness. You can also build exercise into your daily life by choosing to take the stairs instead of the elevator and walking whenever possible. Start wearing a pedometer to record how many steps you take each day—strive for 10,000 per day to start. In addition, you can park farther away from your destination than necessary, take a walk during your lunch hour, or walk the dog for five minutes longer than usual. All of these smaller activities will add up without you even realizing it.

• **Find your groove.** Try out different activities and venues until you figure out the type of exercise (and workout environment) that best meets your specific needs and interests. Some gyms offer free trial memberships, which give you an opportunity to test different equipment and classes before making a monetary commitment. Many classes are "a la carte," so you are not obligated to continue if you do not enjoy the first class. Yoga, pilates, Zumba, kickboxing, body conditioning, interval training, and spin classes are all effective calorie-burning workouts offered at most gyms. We encourage you to try classes that interest you and fit your schedule. For more exercise ideas, refer to the chart of calorie-burning activities on pages 163 to 164.

• **Find an exercise buddy.** Although some people enjoy the "alone time" exercising allows, others find solo workouts to be boring and unmotivating. If you fall into the latter category, recruit a friend, spouse, or family member as an exercise partner. You can schedule days and times to work out together, whether it's walking, running, playing tennis, or a gym session. Exercising with someone else adds a social aspect to physical activity and provides moral support, which will prevent you from dreading your workouts or skipping them altogether. An exercise buddy will also push and challenge you to work harder and longer, and you will do the same for them.

• **Find the fun.** Once in a while, you should change the way you exercise to avoid becoming bored or less motivated. You are more likely to reach your fitness goals and remain dedicated to your workout routine if exercise is fun, so keep it interesting! Plan a weekend hike or bike ride with a group of friends or family members, or walk rather than drive to lunch with a friend. Dance lessons, runners' clubs, and bowling leagues are also great ways to stay in shape without sacrificing fun and variety. If you're technologically savvy, try using the Wii Fit or Wii Sports games. When you think creatively, you're bound to find an activity that suits (and entertains) you.

• **Find the funk.** Studies have shown that most people work out longer and harder when they listen to music. An iPod is a great investment if you don't already own one; if you do, start loading it up with songs that make you want to move. You can even create special workout playlists that consist entirely of energizing songs that pump you up. If "playing that funky music" doesn't do it for you, then try listening to audio books while exercising—anything that holds your interest and energizes you will work.

Everyone has to start somewhere, so don't be discouraged or intimidated by the idea of exercising. Set smaller goals and increase them gradually, as we suggest throughout this journal. Start by walking short distances at a comfortable pace, and once you build your endurance, your slow walk will become more fast-paced until it is eventually a jog or even a run. You will be running 5K races and breezing through hour-long kickboxing classes sooner than you think. If you progress more slowly, however, remember that the important thing is to move and keep moving.

## WEEKLY PERSONAL GOAL

_____

_____

_____

_____

_____

## WEEKLY CONCLUSION

_____

_____

_____

_____

_____

| MONDAY | FOOD | CAL. | | | | H$_2$O |
|---|---|---|---|---|---|---|
| BREAKFAST | | | | | | 🥤 |
| | | | | | | 🥤 |
| | | | | | | 🥤 |

NOTES: _____

| SNACK | | | | | | 🥤 |
|---|---|---|---|---|---|---|
| | | | | | | 🥤 |

NOTES: _____

| LUNCH | | | | | | 🥤 |
|---|---|---|---|---|---|---|
| | | | | | | 🥤 |
| | | | | | | 🥤 |

NOTES: _____

| SNACK | | | | | | 🥤 |
|---|---|---|---|---|---|---|
| | | | | | | 🥤 |

NOTES: _____

| DINNER | | | | | | 🥤 |
|---|---|---|---|---|---|---|
| | | | | | | 🥤 |
| | | | | | | 🥤 |

NOTES: _____

| SNACK | | | | | | 🥤 |
|---|---|---|---|---|---|---|

NOTES: _____

| EXERCISE TYPE | 15 MIN. | 30 MIN. | 45 MIN. | 60 MIN. |
|---|---|---|---|---|
| | | | | |

## TUESDAY

| | FOOD | CAL. | | | | H₂O |
|---|---|---|---|---|---|---|
| **BREAKFAST** | | | | | | 🥤 |
| | | | | | | 🥤 |
| | | | | | | 🥤 |

NOTES: _____

| | | | | | | H₂O |
|---|---|---|---|---|---|---|
| **SNACK** | | | | | | 🥤 |
| | | | | | | 🥤 |

NOTES: _____

| | | | | | | H₂O |
|---|---|---|---|---|---|---|
| **LUNCH** | | | | | | 🥤 |
| | | | | | | 🥤 |
| | | | | | | 🥤 |

NOTES: _____

| | | | | | | H₂O |
|---|---|---|---|---|---|---|
| **SNACK** | | | | | | 🥤 |
| | | | | | | 🥤 |

NOTES: _____

| | | | | | | H₂O |
|---|---|---|---|---|---|---|
| **DINNER** | | | | | | 🥤 |
| | | | | | | 🥤 |
| | | | | | | 🥤 |

NOTES: _____

| | | | | | | |
|---|---|---|---|---|---|---|
| **SNACK** | | | | | | 🥤 |

NOTES: _____

| EXERCISE TYPE | 15 MIN. | 30 MIN. | 45 MIN. | 60 MIN. |
|---|---|---|---|---|
| | | | | |

| WEDNESDAY | FOOD | CAL. | | | | $H_2O$ |
|---|---|---|---|---|---|---|
| BREAKFAST | | | | | | 🥛🥛🥛 |

NOTES:

| SNACK | | | | | | 🥛🥛 |
|---|---|---|---|---|---|---|

NOTES:

| LUNCH | | | | | | 🥛🥛🥛 |
|---|---|---|---|---|---|---|

NOTES:

| SNACK | | | | | | 🥛🥛 |
|---|---|---|---|---|---|---|

NOTES:

| DINNER | | | | | | 🥛🥛🥛 |
|---|---|---|---|---|---|---|

NOTES:

| SNACK | | | | | | 🥛 |
|---|---|---|---|---|---|---|

NOTES:

| EXERCISE TYPE | 15 MIN. | 30 MIN. | 45 MIN. | 60 MIN. |
|---|---|---|---|---|
| | | | | |

# THURSDAY

| FOOD | CAL. | | | | H₂O |
|------|------|---|---|---|-----|

**BREAKFAST**

| | | | | | 🥛 |
|---|---|---|---|---|---|
| | | | | | 🥛 |
| | | | | | 🥛 |

NOTES: _____

**SNACK**

| | | | | | 🥛 |
|---|---|---|---|---|---|
| | | | | | 🥛 |

NOTES: _____

**LUNCH**

| | | | | | 🥛 |
|---|---|---|---|---|---|
| | | | | | 🥛 |
| | | | | | 🥛 |

NOTES: _____

**SNACK**

| | | | | | 🥛 |
|---|---|---|---|---|---|
| | | | | | 🥛 |

NOTES: _____

**DINNER**

| | | | | | 🥛 |
|---|---|---|---|---|---|
| | | | | | 🥛 |
| | | | | | 🥛 |

NOTES: _____

**SNACK**

| | | | | | 🥛 |
|---|---|---|---|---|---|

NOTES: _____

| EXERCISE TYPE | 15 MIN. | 30 MIN. | 45 MIN. | 60 MIN. |
|---------------|---------|---------|---------|---------|
| | | | | |

## FRIDAY

| | FOOD | CAL. | | | | H₂O |
|---|---|---|---|---|---|---|
| **BREAKFAST** | | | | | | 🥤🥤🥤 |
| | | | | | | |
| | | | | | | |
| | | | | | | |

NOTES:

| | FOOD | CAL. | | | | H₂O |
|---|---|---|---|---|---|---|
| **SNACK** | | | | | | 🥤🥤 |
| | | | | | | |

NOTES:

| | FOOD | CAL. | | | | H₂O |
|---|---|---|---|---|---|---|
| **LUNCH** | | | | | | 🥤🥤🥤 |
| | | | | | | |
| | | | | | | |

NOTES:

| | FOOD | CAL. | | | | H₂O |
|---|---|---|---|---|---|---|
| **SNACK** | | | | | | 🥤🥤 |
| | | | | | | |

NOTES:

| | FOOD | CAL. | | | | H₂O |
|---|---|---|---|---|---|---|
| **DINNER** | | | | | | 🥤🥤🥤 |
| | | | | | | |
| | | | | | | |

NOTES:

| | | | | | | H₂O |
|---|---|---|---|---|---|---|
| **SNACK** | | | | | | 🥤 |

NOTES:

| EXERCISE TYPE | 15 MIN. | 30 MIN. | 45 MIN. | 60 MIN. |
|---|---|---|---|---|
| | | | | |

## SATURDAY

| | FOOD | CAL. | | | | H₂O |
|---|---|---|---|---|---|---|
| **BREAKFAST** | | | | | | 🥛 |
| | | | | | | 🥛 |
| | | | | | | 🥛 |
| | | | | | | |

NOTES:

| | | | | | | H₂O |
|---|---|---|---|---|---|---|
| **SNACK** | | | | | | 🥛 |
| | | | | | | 🥛 |

NOTES:

| | | | | | | H₂O |
|---|---|---|---|---|---|---|
| **LUNCH** | | | | | | 🥛 |
| | | | | | | 🥛 |
| | | | | | | 🥛 |
| | | | | | | |

NOTES:

| | | | | | | H₂O |
|---|---|---|---|---|---|---|
| **SNACK** | | | | | | 🥛 |
| | | | | | | 🥛 |

NOTES:

| | | | | | | H₂O |
|---|---|---|---|---|---|---|
| **DINNER** | | | | | | 🥛 |
| | | | | | | 🥛 |
| | | | | | | 🥛 |
| | | | | | | |

NOTES:

| **SNACK** | | | | | 🥛 |
|---|---|---|---|---|---|

NOTES:

| EXERCISE TYPE | 15 MIN. | 30 MIN. | 45 MIN. | 60 MIN. |
|---|---|---|---|---|
| | | | | |

| SUNDAY | FOOD | CAL. | | | | H₂O |
|---|---|---|---|---|---|---|
| BREAKFAST | | | | | | |

NOTES: _____

| SNACK | | | | | | |

NOTES: _____

| LUNCH | | | | | | |

NOTES: _____

| SNACK | | | | | | |

NOTES: _____

| DINNER | | | | | | |

NOTES: _____

| SNACK | | | | | | |

NOTES: _____

| EXERCISE TYPE | | 15 MIN. | 30 MIN. | 45 MIN. | 60 MIN. |
|---|---|---|---|---|---|
| | | | | | |

# Burn, Baby, Burn

If you aren't sure what type of exercise is the most effective, or if you're looking for new workout ideas to vary your routine, we can help. We have compiled a list of the most common forms of exercise, and approximately how many calories you can burn while doing them per hour and half-hour. The calorie amounts below are based on the weights of an average-sized woman and man (140 and 200 pounds, respectively).

## Average Calories Burned in Select Physical Activities

| | CALORIES BURNED IN 30 MINUTES | | CALORIES BURNED IN 1 HOUR | |
|---|---|---|---|---|
| EXERCISE | 140 LBS | 200 LBS | 140 LBS | 200 LBS |
| **Aerobic class** | | | | |
| *Moderate* | 193 | 276 | 386 | 455 |
| *Intense* | 222 | 318 | 455 | 637 |
| **Biking** | | | | |
| *Leisurely* | 126 | 180 | 252 | 360 |
| *Mountain biking* | 268 | 384 | 537 | 768 |
| *Spinning* | 367 | 733 | 740 | 1000+ |
| **Boxing** | | | | |
| *(Punching bag)* | 191 | 381 | 272 | 544 |
| **Elliptical machine** | | | | |
| *Light* | 191 | 382 | 273 | 545 |
| *Moderate* | 286 | 409 | 573 | 818 |
| *Vigorous* | 318 | 455 | 636 | 909 |
| **Hiking** | 202 | 288 | 403 | 576 |
| **Pilates** | 140 | 222 | 159 | 318 |

| EXERCISE | CALORIES BURNED IN 30 MINUTES | | CALORIES BURNED IN 1 HOUR | |
|---|---|---|---|---|
| | **140 LBS** | **200 LBS** | **140 LBS** | **200 LBS** |
| **Playing with kids** *(Moderate to high level of activity)* | 126 | 180 | 252 | 360 |
| **Pushing a stroller** | 84 | 120 | 186 | 240 |
| **Running** | | | | |
| *8-minute mile* | 397 | 567 | 794 | 1135 |
| *9-minute mile* | 349 | 499 | 699 | 998 |
| *10-minute mile* | 333 | 476 | 667 | 953 |
| **Stair-climbing machine** *(Moderate intensity)* | 286 | 408 | 572 | 816 |
| **Swimming** | | | | |
| *Leisurely* | 202 | 288 | 403 | 576 |
| *Vigorous* | 310 | 443 | 621 | 819 |
| **Tennis** | | | | |
| *Singles* | 193 | 276 | 386 | 364 |
| *Doubles* | 134 | 192 | 268 | 384 |
| **Walking** *(3.5 miles/hour)* | 134 | 192 | 269 | 384 |
| **Weight training** | | | | |
| *Moderate* | 109 | 156 | 218 | 346 |
| *Vigorous* | 193 | 276 | 386 | 552 |
| **Wii Fit** | | | | |
| *Beginner* | 78 | 114 | 156 | 228 |
| *Advanced* | 109 | 161 | 217 | 322 |
| **Wii Boxing** | 162 | 252 | 324 | 504 |
| **Yoga** *(Hatha)* | 79 | 113 | 159 | 227 |
| **Zumba** | 175–250 | 250–400 | 350–500 | 500–800 |

# Conclusion

## Maintaining Your Healthy New Life

Congratulations! You have completed our ten-week *Bite It and Write It* program, hopefully with more successes than struggles. We hope that this journal has made you more aware of your old eating habits and inspired you to develop new ones. We also hope that keeping a food log and striving towards our weekly goals has given you a new perspective on nutritional wellness. Above all, we hope that *Bite It and Write It* has steered you in the direction of true lifestyle change.

As you now know, it all starts with *writing it down*. Keeping track of what you eat is the first step in becoming a healthy and mindful eater. You have taken this step, and now, ten weeks later, you are equipped with invaluable nutritional knowledge; more importantly, you are equipped with invaluable *self*-knowledge. You know now what you are capable of, and you have undoubtedly noticed a difference in how you look and feel—what tastes better than that? Nothing!

But it does not end here. The next step is just as important: Maintain the self-discipline, nutrition, and fitness that you have practiced over the past ten weeks. We encourage you to start another journal so you can continue a structured food log. Alternatively, begin keeping track of your eating, drinking, and workout habits in a notebook. Always remember that you are not alone in this process; there are plenty of professionals you can speak to and support websites you can join. Enlist the help of family and friends— they will be a great source of moral support and encouragement for you. The more support you get, the better off you will be.

Ultimately, however, the rest is up to *you*. You are the only person who can truly make you eat right, move more, and fully commit to a healthier life. All it takes is knowledge and dedication. This journal has given you the knowledge, so now you have the power to dedicate yourself to a healthier you.

# Appendix A

## CALORIE GUIDE FOR COMMON FOODS

The following pages are your calorie guide for commonly consumed foods. We have provided this mini-calorie counter so that you can always look up certain foods and drinks in order to make an informed and healthy choice, and control your calorie intake at almost every meal, every day.

### CALORIE GUIDE TO COMMON FOODS

| FOOD DESCRIPTION | AMOUNT | CALORIES |
|---|---|---|
| **ALCOHOL** | | |
| Beer, regular | 12 oz. | 150 |
| Beer, light | 12 oz. | 100 |
| Beer, extra light | 12 oz. | 75 |
| Champagne | 6 oz. | 128 |
| Frozen Margarita | 6.5 oz. | 245 |
| Gin and Tonic<br>(2 oz. gin, 4 oz. tonic) | 6 oz. | 175 |
| LIQUOR<br>(Gin, Rum, Tequila, Vodka,<br>or Whiskey, 80 Proof ) | 1.5 oz. | 100 |
| Martini w/ Vermouth<br>and 1 Olive | 2.5 oz. | 184 |

| | | |
|---|---|---|
| Vodka w/ Cranberry Juice (1.5 oz. vodka, 4.5 oz. cranberry juice) | 6 oz. | 172 |
| Wine, Red | 6 oz. | 128 |
| Wine, Sweet Riesling | 6 oz. | 270 |
| Wine, White | 6 oz. | 120 |

## BEVERAGES (NON-ALCOHOLIC)

| | | |
|---|---|---|
| Caffe Latte, non-fat | 12 oz. | 110 |
| Cappuccino, non-fat | 12 oz. | 75 |
| Coffee, black | 8 oz. | 4 |
| Fruit Juice | 8 oz. | 110 |
| Iced Tea, sweetened | 8 oz. | 70 |
| Soft Drinks | 8 oz. | 110 |
| Soft Drinks | 12 oz. | 140 |
| Tea, Black or Green | 8 oz. | 2 |
| Water | any amount | 0 |

## TEA/COFFEE ADDITIONS

| | | |
|---|---|---|
| Cream, half and half | 2 tbsp. | 40 |
| Cream, light | 2 tbsp. | 60 |
| Creamer, liquid | 2 tbsp. | 40 |
| Creamer, powdered | 2 tbsp. | 20 |
| Milk, low-fat | 2 tbsp. | 15 |
| Milk, non-fat | 2 tbsp. | 10 |
| Milk, whole | 2 tbsp. | 20 |

## MILK AND MILK SUBSTITUTES

| | | |
|---|---|---|
| Almond Milk | 8 oz. | 40 |
| Coconut Milk | 8 oz. | 50 |
| Cow's Milk, whole | 8 oz. | 150 |
| Cow's Milk, 2% | 8 oz. | 130 |
| Cow's Milk, 1% | 8 oz. | 110 |

## MILK AND MILK SUBSTITUTES (CONTINUED)

| | | |
|---|---|---|
| Cow's Milk, fat-free | 8 oz. | 90 |
| Soy Milk | 8 oz. | 130 |
| Soy Milk, light | 8 oz. | 80 |

## BREADS, WRAPS, & GRAINS

| | | |
|---|---|---|
| Bagel, plain | 1 (3.2 oz.) | 300 |
| Bagel, whole wheat | 1 (3.2 oz.) | 300 |
| Bread, whole wheat | 1 slice | 90 |
| Bun, whole wheat | 1 | 100 |
| Barley | 1 cup | 200 |
| Couscous | 3/4 cup | 200 |
| Pasta, white | 1 cup | 220 |
| Pasta, whole grain | 1 cup | 220 |
| Pita, whole wheat (small) | 1 | 100 |
| Pita, whole wheat (large) | 1 | 200 |
| Quinoa, cooked | 1 cup | 290 |
| Rice, brown | 1 cup | 200 |
| Rice, white | 1 cup | 200 |
| Wheat Berries | 1 cup | 220 |
| Wrap, plain (small) | 1 | 90 |
| Wrap, plain (large) | 1 | 180 |

## BREAKFAST CEREALS

| | | |
|---|---|---|
| All Bran | ½ cup | 80 |
| Barbara's Puffins | ¾ cup | 90 |
| Barbara's Shredded Spoonfuls | ¾ cup | 120 |
| Bare Naked Granola | ¼ cup | 100 |
| Cascadian Farm Hearty Morning Fiber | ¾ cup | 200 |
| Cheerios | 1 cup | 110 |
| Kashi Go Lean | 1 cup | 140 |
| Kashi Heart To Heart | ¾ cup | 110 |

## BREAKFAST CEREALS (CONTINUED)

| | | |
|---|---|---|
| Kashi Whole Grain Flakes | 1 cup | 180 |
| Nature's Path Smart Bran | ⅔ cup | 90 |
| Oatmeal, plain (cooked) | ½ cup | 100 |
| Raisin Bran | 1 cup | 190 |
| Simply Fiber | 1 cup | 100 |

## CONDIMENTS & SPREADS

| | | |
|---|---|---|
| Agave | 1 tbsp. | 60 |
| Almond Butter | 2 tbsp. | 200 |
| BBQ Sauce | 1 tbsp. | 50 |
| Cocktail Sauce | 1 tbsp. | 30 |
| Guacamole | ¼ cup | 43 |
| Honey | 1 tbsp. | 60 |
| Hummus | 2 tbsp. | 25 |
| Jelly, Jam, & Preserves | 1 tbsp. | 50 |
| Ketchup | 1 packet | 20 |
| Peanut Butter | 2 tbsp. | 190 |

## DAIRY PRODUCTS
### Cheese

| | | |
|---|---|---|
| American Cheese | 1 slice | 110 |
| Cheese, 2% (average brand) | 1 oz. | 80 |
| Cottage Cheese, creamed | 1 cup | 230 |
| Cottage Cheese, low-fat | 1 cup | 200 |
| Cottage Cheese, non-fat | 1 cup | 150 |
| Farmer's Cheese | 2 tbsp. | 40 |
| Feta Cheese, reduced fat | ¼ cup | 70 |
| Feta Cheese, whole | ¼ cup | 90 |
| Goat Cheese | ¼ cup | 110 |
| Gorgonzola/Bleu Cheese | ¼ cup | 110 |
| Hard Cheese | 1 oz. | 115 |
| Mozzarella Cheese, part skim | 1 oz. | 72 |
| Mozzarella Cheese, whole | 1 oz. | 90 |

**Eggs**

| | | |
|---|---|---|
| Large | 1 | 75 |
| Large, fried | 1 | 105 |
| Omelet | 2 | 190 |
| Omelet, egg whites only | 4 | 80 |
| Whites only | 1 | 20 |
| Egg Salad (2 eggs, 1 tbsp. mayo) | 3 oz. | 253 |
| Egg Salad (2 eggs, 2 tbsp. mayo) | 3.2 oz. | 340 |

**Yogurt**

| | | |
|---|---|---|
| Plain, fat-free | 1 cup | 130 |
| Plain Greek Yogurt (2%) | 1 cup | 140 |
| Plain Greek Yogurt (0%) | 1 cup | 100 |
| Flavored/Fruit, fat-free | 1 cup | 80 |
| Flavored/Fruit, low-fat | 1 cup | 215 |
| Flavored/Fruit, whole | 1 cup | 230 |

**FATS AND OILS**

| | | |
|---|---|---|
| Butter, regular | 1 tbsp. | 102 |
| Butter, whipped | 1 tbsp. | 75 |
| Margarine, light | 1 tbsp. | 50 |
| Margarine, regular | 1 tbsp. | 75 |
| Oil & Vinegar | 1 tbsp. | 55 |
| Oils | 1 tbsp. | 110 |
| Vinegar | 1 tbsp. | 0 |
| Ranch Salad Dressing | 1 tbsp. | 80 |

**FISH**

| | | |
|---|---|---|
| Flounder, Sole | 4 oz. | 135 |
| Halibut | 4 oz. | 160 |
| Lox/Nova | 3 oz. | 99 |

**FISH (CONTINUED)**

| | | |
|---|---|---|
| Orange Roughy | 4 oz. | 190 |
| Salmon | 4 oz. | 200 |
| Sardines | 1 cup | 300 |
| Shrimp | 4 oz. | 145 |
| Tuna | 4 oz. | 160 |
| Tuna Fish (1 tbsp. mayo) | 3 oz. | 192 |
| Tuna Fish (2 tbsp. mayo) | 3 oz. | 380 |
| Tuna Salad | 4 oz. | 300 |
| Tuna Salad, light | 4 oz. | 210 |

**FROZEN TREATS**

| | | |
|---|---|---|
| Edy's Frozen Fruit Bars | 1 bar | 70 |
| Häagen-Dazs Cookies & Cream | ½ cup | 270 |
| Skinny Cow Pops | 1 pop | 100 |
| Sorbet | ½ cup | 120 |
| Tofutti Frozen Dessert | ½ cup | 190 |
| Vanilla Ice Cream, light | ½ cup | 140 |
| Vanilla Frozen Yogurt | ½ cup | 120 |

**FRUIT**

| | | |
|---|---|---|
| Apple, medium | 5.5 oz. | 80 |
| Apricot | 1 | 17 |
| Avocado | 1 oz. or 3 slices | 50 |
| Avocado, medium | ½ | 140 |
| Banana, small or medium | 1 | 90–105 |
| Berries | 1 cup | 60 |
| Cherries | 1 cup | 90 |
| Grapefruit, large | ½ cup | 55 |
| Grapes | 1 cup | 60 |
| Kiwi, sliced | 1 cup | 110 |

## FRUIT (CONTINUED)

| | | |
|---|---|---|
| Mango | 1 cup | 110 |
| Melon | 1 cup | 60 |
| Nectarine, medium | 5.3 oz. | 60 |
| Orange, medium | 1 | 70 |
| Papaya | 1 cup | 55 |
| Peach, medium | 5.3 oz. | 60 |
| Pear, medium Bosc | 1 cup | 100 |
| Pineapple, diced | 1 cup | 75 |
| Plum, medium | 1 | 40 |
| Watermelon | 2 cups | 90 |

## MEAT & POULTRY

| | | |
|---|---|---|
| Applegate Farms Chicken | 3 oz. | 80 |
| Applegate Farms Ham | 3 oz. | 80 |
| Applegate Farms Turkey | 3 oz. | 80 |
| Applegate Farms Turkey Hotdog | 1 | 80 |
| Chicken Breast, no skin | 3 oz. | 145 |
| Chicken Thigh, no skin | 3 oz. | 178 |
| Chicken/Turkey Sausage | 1 | 120 |
| Ground Beef, 93% lean | 4 oz. | 170 |
| Ground Turkey, 93% lean | 4 oz. | 160 |
| London Broil | 3 oz. | 210 |
| Pork Chops, boneless | 4 oz. | 160 |
| Prime Rib | 3 oz. | 240 |
| Roast Beef, extra lean | 3 oz. | 90 |
| Sirloin Steak | 3 oz. | 166 |

## NUTS, SEEDS, & LEGUMES

| | | |
|---|---|---|
| Almonds | 1 oz. | 162 |
| Cannellini | ½ cup | 120 |
| Chickpeas (Garbanzo beans) | ½ cup | 142 |

## NUTS, SEEDS, & LEGUMES (CONTINUED)

| | | |
|---|---|---|
| Edamame | ½ cup | 141 |
| Flaxseeds, ground | 1 tbsp. | 37 |
| Kidney Beans | ½ cup | 26 |
| Lentils | ½ cup | 115 |
| Pumpkin Seeds | 1 oz. | 126 |
| Sunflower Seeds | 1 oz. | 165 |

## VEGETABLES

| | | |
|---|---|---|
| Acorn Squash, cubed | 1 cup | 56 |
| Asparagus, raw | 1 cup/10 stalks | 27 |
| Beets | 1 cup | 58 |
| Black Beans | ½ cup | 90 |
| Broccoli, raw | 1 cup | 31 |
| Cabbage, cooked | ½ cup | 17 |
| Carrots (Baby), raw | 1 cup | 50 |
| Cauliflower, raw | 1 cup | 25 |
| Corn | ½ ear | 80 |
| Green Beans, steamed | ½ cup | 20 |
| Lettuce | 1 cup | 10 |
| Onions, chopped | 1 cup | 32 |
| Pepper (Bell), medium | 1 | 30 |
| Potato, baked (no skin), medium | 1 or 5 oz. | 145 |
| Potato, Sweet | 1 cup | 180 |
| Scallions, chopped | 1 cup | 32 |
| Tomato, Grape | 1 cup | 30 |
| Tomato, medium | 1 | 22 |
| Zucchini, chopped | 1 cup | 20 |

# Appendix B

## CALORIE GUIDE FOR CHAIN RESTAURANT FOODS

Considering the regularity with which people go out to eat nowadays, a calorie guide wouldn't be complete without a list of calorie information for the most commonly frequented restaurants. We strongly suggest that you use this calorie counter to help you make smart choices when dining out, but be aware that this guide is only a sampling of the options available at these restaurants. If there is a chain restaurant that you eat at on a regular basis that does not appear on this list, or if we have not included a particular meal you usually order, take a few minutes to look for nutritional data on their website. What you learn may convince you to choose your meals more carefully and healthfully.

### CALORIE GUIDE TO COMMONLY FREQUENTED RESTAURANTS

| CALIFORNIA PIZZA KITCHEN | |
| --- | --- |
| **FOOD** | **CALORIES** |
| BBQ Chopped Chicken Salad with Avocado, full | 1,257 |
| Chinese Chicken Salad, full | 707 |
| Grilled Vegetable Salad with Chicken, full | 1,044 |

| | |
|---|---|
| Pizza, Five Cheese and Tomato | 1,114 |
| Pizza, Hawaiian BBQ Chicken | 1,159 |
| Pizza, Kids | 425 |
| Soup, Asparagus (bowl) | 213 |
| Soup, White Bean Minestrone (bowl) | 245 |

## COSI

| FOOD | CALORIES |
|---|---|
| Grilled Chicken TBM Sandwich | 691 |
| Grilled Chicken TBM Sandwich, Lighter Side | 531 |
| Hummus & Fresh Veggies Sandwich | 397 |
| Pesto Chicken Melt | 671 |
| Pizza, Pepperoni | 806 |
| Pizza, Traditional | 883 |
| Roasted Turkey & Brie Sandwich | 687 |
| Salad, Cobb Light | 519 |
| Salad, Signature Light | 371 |
| Tuna Melt | 874 |
| Tuna Sandwich | 539 |
| Turkey Light Sandwich | 390 |

## DUNKIN DONUTS

| BEVERAGES | CALORIES |
|---|---|
| Cappuccino, small | 80 |
| Coffee Coolatta, small (skim milk) | 210 |
| Hot Chocolate, small | 230 |
| Iced Cappuccino, light, medium | 40 |
| Iced Tea, sweetened, small | 80 |
| Latte, small | 120 |
| Latte, Mocha Raspberry, small | 23 |

| FOOD | CALORIES |
| --- | --- |
| Bagel, Plain | 320 |
| Bagel, Multigrain | 390 |
| Bran Muffin | 450 |
| Cream Cheese, reduced fat (1 serving) | 100 |
| Cream Cheese, regular (1 serving) | 150 |
| Croissant, Plain | 310 |
| Donut, Glazed | 220 |
| Donut, Jelly or Créme-Filled | 260–280 |
| Egg & Cheese on English Muffin (DD Smart) | 320 |
| Egg White & Cheese on English Muffin (DD Smart) | 270 |
| Egg White Veggie Flatbread | 290 |
| Ham, Egg, & Cheese on Bagel | 510 |
| Munchkins | 50–60 per Munchkin |

## MCDONALD'S

| FOOD | CALORIES |
| --- | --- |
| Big Mac | 540 |
| Cheeseburger | 300 |
| Chicken Nuggets (10 pieces) | 420 |
| Chicken Select, large order | 630 |
| Egg McMuffin | 300 |
| French Fries, small order | 250 |
| Fruit & Yogurt Parfait | 160 |
| Hamburger | 250 |
| Hot Cakes w/ 2 pats margarine and syrup | 610 |
| McChicken Sandwich | 360 |
| Vanilla Shake, small | 420 |

## MOE'S

| FOOD | CALORIES |
| --- | --- |
| Billy Barou Chicken Nachos (all toppings) | 1,495 |

| | |
|---|---:|
| Close Talker, Salad with Chicken, Black Beans, and Guacamole (no shell or cheese) | 388 |
| Close Talker, Salad with Chicken, Black Beans, Cheese, and Crispy Salad Bowl (no guacamole) | 795 |
| Fat Sam, Steak Fajita (all toppings) | 1,078 |
| Fat Sam, Steak Fajita (no cheese or sour cream) | 768 |
| Homewrecker with Chicken (all toppings) | 925 |
| John Coctosan, Chicken & Cheese Quesadilla (no sour cream) | 680 |
| Overachiever, Hard-Shell Beef Taco (all toppings) | 345 |

## PANERA BREAD

| FOOD | CALORIES |
|---|---:|
| Asiago Roast Beef on Asiago Cheese Bread, full | 690 |
| Asian Sesame Chicken Salad, full | 400 |
| Bacon, Egg, & Cheese on Ciabatta Bread | 510 |
| Chicken Caesar Salad, full | 510 |
| Chicken Caesar on Three Cheese Bread, full | 710 |
| Chopped Chicken Cobb Salad, full | 500 |
| Cinnamon Roll | 620 |
| Egg & Cheese on Ciabatta Bread | 380 |
| Frontega Chicken Hot Panini, full | 860 |
| Italian Combo on Ciabatta Bread, full | 1,040 |
| Mac & Cheese, small | 490 |
| Mediterranean Chicken Salad, full | 480 |
| Napa Almond Chicken Salad Sandwich, full | 680 |
| Sierra Turkey on Foccacia Bread with Asiago Cheese Bread, full | 970 |
| Strawberry Granola Parfait | 280 |

## STARBUCKS

| BEVERAGES | CALORIES |
|---|---|
| Cappuccino, Grande (2% milk) | 230 |
| Caramel Macchiato, Tall | 240 |
| Frappuccino, Grande (2% milk) | 230 |
| Frappuccino, Tazo Green Tea Crème, Tall (2% milk) | 310 |
| Latte, Grande (2% milk) | 190 |
| Skinny Iced Coffee, Tall | 25 |
| Skinny Latte, Flavored, Grande (2% milk) | 180 |
| Skinny Tazo Awake Tea Latte | 80 |
| Tazo Iced Passion Tea, unsweetened | 0 |

| FOOD | CALORIES |
|---|---|
| 8-Grain Roll | 350 |
| Coffeecake, Starbucks Classic | 440 |
| Cookie, Chocolate Chunk | 360 |
| Cookie, Outrageous Oatmeal | 370 |
| Marshmallow Dream Bar | 210 |
| Muffin, Low-Fat Raspberry | 340 |
| Muffin, Zucchini Walnut | 490 |
| Panini, Tuna Melt | 390 |
| Sandwich, Ham & Swiss | 360 |
| Sandwich, Turkey & Swiss | 390 |
| Wrap, Chicken & Vegetable | 290 |

# About the Authors

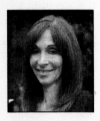

*Stacie Castle, MS, RD, CDN*, received her BS degree in Food and Nutrition from Queens College, CUNY, and her Masters degree in Public Health Nutrition from Columbia University. She honed her counseling and clinical skills as she worked in health clubs and a prestigious long-term care facility, where she was one of the first dietitians in New York City to define the role of a nutritionist within a Long-Term Home Health Care Program. Stacie opened her own practice in 2001 in Lake Success, New York, where she counsels and inspires thousands of people with type 2 diabetes, insulin resistance, obesity, celiac disease, and gastrointestinal and metabolic issues. She also offers worksite nutrition lectures to corporations and non-profit agencies. In the fall of 2009, Stacie successfully passed the American Dietetic Association course to obtain a Certification of Training in Adult Weight Management. By using motivational counseling techniques, Stacie has come to know the powerful effects food can have in the prevention and management of disease.

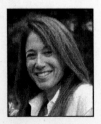

*Robyn A. Cotler, MS, RD, CDN*, received her BS degree from University of Maryland and her Masters in Clinical Nutrition from New York University, where she also completed her internship. Robyn has coauthored a research paper with Rockefeller University Hospital on diet's influence on blood cholesterol, and has written for *Woodbury Magazine* and several other newsletters. As a regular guest speaker for elementary and middle school students, she has influenced children to make better food choices. In addition, she has been a guest speaker for cancer and bariatric support groups. Robyn continues to practice in the Woodbury/Plainview area providing individual nutritional recommendations for diabetes, gastric bariatric surgery, family nutrition, and celiac disease.

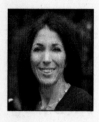

*Marni Schefter, RD, CDN,* graduated from the University of Michigan, Ann Arbor. She completed her dietetic internship at the C.W. Post Campus of Long Island University, and her last rotation was at North Shore University Hospital in Manhasset, New York, where she continued as a clinical dietitian. For the next three years, Marni simultaneously worked at North Shore and counseled clients out of the private practice she opened in Wantagh, New York, and she continues to offer counseling in weight control, hyperlipidemia, diabetes, eating disorders, and sports nutrition at her Wantagh office. Marni is an active member of the American Dietetic Association and the Long Island Diet Association, for which she chaired a private practice reimbursement committee. In addition to serving as a consultant to various eating establishments on Long Island, Marni gives lectures to classes and audiences at private restaurants.

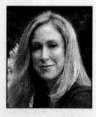

*Shana Shapiro, MS, RD, CDN, CDE,* received her BS degree in psychology from Emory University and her Masters in Nutrition Education from Teacher's College at Columbia University. She completed her internship at New York Presbyterian Medical

Center and continued her career as a registered dietitian there for the next five years, specializing in cardiovascular disease and diabetes. Shana has had the pleasure of treating Dr. Mehmet Oz's patients and working closely with the Naomi Berrie Diabetes Center, and her work at the hospital led her to become a Certified Diabetes Educator. Currently, Shana maintains a successful private practice in Roslyn Heights, New York, that specializes in weight management, medical nutrition therapy, and family wellness. In addition to counseling patients, she lectures to a variety of audiences including students, support groups, and the general public.

To learn more about the authors and their work in nutrition:

**Website:** www.biteitandwriteit.com
**Twitter:** @biteitnwriteit
**Facebook:** biteitandwriteit
**Email:** biteitandwriteit@gmail.com